THE **MODERN MIDWIFE'S** GUIDE TO

THE FIRST YEAR

Also by Marie Louise

The Modern Midwife's Guide to Pregnancy, Birth and Beyond

THE MODERN MIDWIFE'S GUIDE TO
THE FIRST YEAR

Marie Louise

1

Vermilion, an imprint of Ebury Publishing
20 Vauxhall Bridge Road
London SW1V 2SA

Vermilion is part of the Penguin Random House group of companies
whose addresses can be found at global.penguinrandomhouse.com

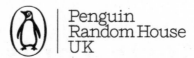

Copyright © Marie Louise 2023

Illustrations by Hannah Fleetwood

Marie Louise has asserted her right to be identified as the author of this
Work in accordance with the Copyright, Designs and Patents Act 1988

First published by Vermilion in 2023

www.penguin.co.uk

A CIP catalogue record for this book is available from the British Library

ISBN 9781785044113

Typeset in 10/13.5 pt FuturaBT by Jouve (UK), Milton Keynes
Printed and bound in Great Britain by Clays Ltd, Elcograf S.p.A.

The authorised representative in the EEA is Penguin Random House Ireland,
Morrison Chambers, 32 Nassau Street, Dublin D02 YH68

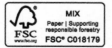

MIX
Paper | Supporting
responsible forestry
FSC® C018179

Penguin Random House is committed to a
sustainable future for our business, our readers
and our planet. This book is made from Forest
Stewardship Council® certified paper.

CONTENTS

~~~~~

Introduction

WELCOME TO THE wonderful world of motherhood. If you're reading this, I am sure you've already been on a huge journey and are about to embark on another one – the first year of your baby's life. You may be reading this book during pregnancy, shortly after birth or several months later. Wherever you are on your journey, it's great that you're here – feel free to dip in and out of the book as you need to.

Becoming someone's mother is one of the greatest and hardest transformations life has to offer. We are all unique individuals and there's never one way of doing anything. Yet there are many questions, decisions and opinions. It can be really tough for new mums to know who to take advice from, where they fit in within mum groups, and to settle into themselves as mothers. You are a different person after becoming a mum. There are many changes within the first year and I want you to know now that if you find this hard at times it's because motherhood, whether it's for the first or fifth time, *is* hard. Especially in today's world with all its pressures on so many areas of our lives – from social media and careers to our identity. More often than not, you can trust your gut instinct to guide you, especially once you build confidence as a mother.

As a midwife for many years, I assumed I would cope with motherhood well. I thought I knew what I was doing, at least at the beginning. I thought motherhood would come naturally to me and I would be able to trust my intuition and instincts as a mum. Part of this was true, but much of it never really became reality. My intuition seemed to get lost in my emotions, self-doubt crept in and it was hard to think straight. At times I didn't know who to listen to or even the best place to turn. Some of those difficulties are normal, such as the extreme emotions you feel, and may serve a purpose, but the confusion and self-doubt can be mitigated with the right support, science and a little guidance. Eventually I managed to reach a healthy balance of being able to listen to advice and pick what I wanted to take away and what I wanted to leave.

My aim in this book is to offer you some guidance during the first year of your baby's life and your life as a new mum. I have highlighted what to expect at different times, with a constant yet important reminder that all babies are different and you will know what's right for yours. When I wrote my first book – *The Modern Midwife's Guide to Pregnancy, Birth and Beyond* – I had not had a baby. Now that I have joined you and become a mother to the absolute love of my life, Georgie, I am able to share some of my own experiences as well as offer you support that is backed by research. Along the way you'll find 'honesty boxes' where I have shared some deeply personal experiences which I hope you'll find helpful. I have purposely chosen not to sugar-coat things because I think real-life experiences and raw emotions help mothers more than glossing over or making light of a tough situation. Your journey will be unique and different to mine, but I'm sure you'll find yourself nodding along in agreement in a few places. I hope you find comfort in knowing you're not alone. Writing about my emotions and difficulties has been a healing experience. I laughed and cried many times, and I thought of you reading this and how amazing we parents really are.

You deserve to feel confident and better able to care for yourself as well as your baby, and I hope this book enables you to do just that. There's a lot to cover and a lot to talk about, as ever so much happens within that first year: from recovering from birth, to teething, weaning and sleeping, to supporting your baby to learn and develop (their brain doubles in weight within the first year of life), your relationship, if you are in one, and then you, mama. It is going to be okay.

We cover each section chronologically. Take it slow and try not to think too much about how you'll cope with the next phase. Some light planning and awareness will do, but focusing on what's happening now, in the present moment, may be best; we can often overthink things as mums or beat ourselves up if we don't get it 'right'. We all make mistakes and we learn – motherhood is all about adapting and learning on the job, so to speak. Whether this is your first baby or not, all babies are different and come with their individual ways.

Throughout our journey through the first year I have a few experts joining us. I am an experienced midwife and mum, but my main expertise is within the first eight weeks after birth. That's why, as well as incorporating my own research, I have discussed different areas relevant to you with experts I trust or who have personally helped me.

HOW TO USE THIS BOOK

~~~~~

To keep it simple, I have divided the book into parts based on three-month intervals, the exception being the first part, where we focus on the initial 48 hours – this time warrants a separate section, as I hope you'll agree after reading through it:

- The first 48 hours after birth
- Newborn to three months
- Three to six months
- Six to nine months
- Nine to twelve months

This book is a natural progression from my first book and I hope you find it just as supportive and nurturing, which is an intention I always set out with when I start writing. There are inevitably a few crossovers between the two books in a couple of places, but if you would like to know more about pregnancy and birth, please do have a look at my first book which is full of information about these topics. Once again, you'll find key points at the end of each section. Mums are super-busy and I appreciate you may not always have time to read the whole section, so the key takeaways are there to help set reminders. You may also want to use them as a prompt, to see if that section is relevant to you at the time.

Because many of my readers highlighted these key points as a helpful tool in my first book, I wanted to expand on them here and thought you might find a special section with my top tips helpful too (see pages 235–40). These are little bits of information I have gleaned along the way, notes to myself and quick reminders. This section is intended to support you to take what you find helpful and leave anything that doesn't feel authentic to you. We all have different ways of approaching the same situation and that's okay. I hope you find something helpful in and among those tips to implement on your journey.

There's also a final note to you on page 233. You may want to come back to this and read it if you're having a tough time, or difficulty crossing from one stage to the next and need some reassurance or a reminder.

No matter what happens on your journey through motherhood you will learn that you're stronger than you ever knew, and that sometimes the toughest times lead to real personal growth and make you a better version of yourself. Watching your baby grow and learn about the wonders of the world is one of the most beautiful miracles life has to offer. This is such an exciting and huge chapter in your life.

You've got this! x

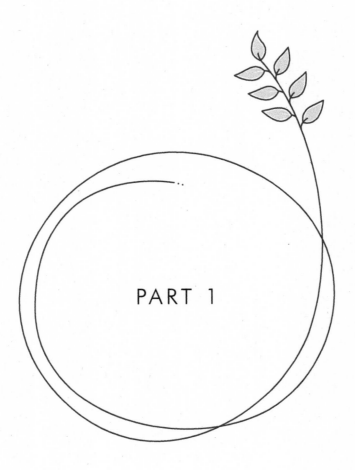

PART 1

The First 48 Hours After Birth

A very warm welcome to the wonderful world of motherhood, mama. In the early hours after birth, feelings are difficult to put into words and are likely to be bigger than you ever could have imagined. This is very normal for all mums. You've just experienced one of the biggest events life has to offer. Allow yourself to go through all of these powerful emotions: the scary love, worry, tiredness, amazement, vulnerability, pride, relief, fear . . . (I'm sure you've got a few more to add).

The first 48 hours will look different for everyone and depend on a few things, such as the type of birth you had, what happened during the birth and immediately after, who was with you, where you gave birth, how many weeks your baby was born at, and how well you are both recovering from the birth. These will all be unique to you and your new baby. In addition, there are so many aspects that have an effect on your individual experience – your birth experience, any medication you had, and the length of your labour, to name a few. There's no right or wrong way to feel. Some mums get that instant rush of love; others don't. There's nothing wrong with you if you don't get this right away. Your birth experience will impact those very early feelings and emotions. If your experience differs greatly from what you were expecting or had heard about, this may make you feel alone. I can absolutely *promise you* that someone somewhere in the world is experiencing exactly the same situation as you.

In this part we are going to start with some of the things you may experience soon after birth, including the clinical checks and wound care. We'll then move on to birth experiences and how to manage them. We will run through a few types of experiences and hopefully you will finish this section with more understanding of why you may feel a certain way and have confidence to ask questions. Lastly, the focus shifts to your newborn baby, starting with caring for their skin and cord, initiating breastfeeding, normal newborn behaviour, and the role of healthcare professionals – once you're home. I've created a little list of places and organisations you may find helpful in the resources section on page 241.

Whether you're a first-time mum or have given birth several times before, this will be a new experience and will change your family dynamic. It's important to know from the start, *this* early on in your journey, that there will be things that throw you, make you feel vulnerable, and you may even question everything you thought you knew about yourself. All mums go through a huge transitional phase and transformation when they have a new baby. It's going to be okay. You'll work through the hard times and you will be an amazing mum. In these first 48 hours I'd really recommend you carefully carve out some protected time for yourself and time to bond with your baby – uninterrupted. For those of you with babies in the special care baby unit (also know as SCBU or NICU), you can still recreate this bonding time once your baby is ready. You haven't missed out – it's a little delayed perhaps, but you'll have this moment and it will be blissful.

Clinical observations post-birth

WHEN YOU ARE moved to the postnatal ward, or if you are being discharged home from a midwifery-led unit, the first check you can expect during the postnatal care pathway is often referred to as a 'full postnatal check'. It is a thorough top-to-toe assessment of you. At the same time your baby will receive a 'neonatal check' – should you consent to these, of course. Your midwives will document everything in a checklist-style table either on paper or digitally, depending on whether or not the hospital you receive care from has gone paperless.

After taking into account the type of birth you had and any additional concerns or risk factors (most commonly due to infection, meconium, blood loss or any complications during pregnancy), you may be offered more frequent checks or blood tests. If this is the case, it is important to ask all the questions you have so that you can make an informed choice about whether or not you would like to accept the recommendations or tests. I want to be really clear here: I am not suggesting you decline recommendations from your healthcare providers. Instead, I am encouraging you to ask questions to ensure you have a full understanding of what is happening medically and why. We all have different perceptions of risk and the hospital may have a particular policy due to extensive research and reliable statistics, a previous case that led to a poor outcome, or a clinician's expert opinion. That does not mean to say that their risk assessment is in line with yours or that you have to do or administer anything to yourself or your baby that does not seem appropriate to you. Only you can decide what you think is necessary. And you won't be able to make that judgement until you ask those questions. That said, some people are happy to follow every recommendation because following all recommendations is what makes them feel safe. We are all very different – whatever works best for you is fine.

'HOW ARE YOU?'

~~~~

Your midwife will likely start by asking you how you are feeling. Speaking to you directly is the number one way many clinicians assess your individual needs, so please give your midwife as much information as possible and always be honest. So many mums say 'fine' when I ask this. It's okay not to feel fine and it's best to let your midwife know if that is the case so they can really support you to heal or address any of the concerns you have. The majority of further tests or diagnoses I have made in my career usually start with what a woman tells me, not by completing my checklist. That's not to discredit the list – it's helpful when you have a lot to remember – but the information you tell us takes priority. You're the expert when it comes to your own body and you know when you don't feel right. Please use this question to address *any* concerns you have about yourself. And try to focus on yourself here. The number of times mums reply with something like, 'So, the baby wouldn't settle in the cot last night . . .' Yes, it's important we address every concern and question you have about your baby, but try to think about your needs here. Even just for that one question, your health, healing and wellbeing matter.

OBSERVATIONS AND ADDITIONAL TESTS

~~~~

After your midwife has covered your concerns, answered questions or concluded whether you need further tests/referrals, they will undertake a full set of clinical observations – this is nothing out of the ordinary so try not to worry. Generally, that's your blood pressure, heart rate, respiratory rate and temperature. If you're in hospital or have had a heavier bleed, your midwife may want to check your oxygen saturation levels too. There are some additional checks or blood tests that you might be offered, but that is completely dependent on any current medical condition and symptoms. You should also be asked about your breasts, whether you are breastfeeding or not. Don't hesitate to remind your midwife or doctor of any follow-up tests that have previously been recommended to you. It's unlikely these will be missed, but it's always good to ensure there's good communication and that your expectations surrounding what was to come are in alignment with what is being recommended/undertaken.

WOUNDS AND BLEEDING

~~~~~

Once the observations have been taken, next they will want to assess any wounds, either from a C-section or due to perineal trauma – we'll go into more detail about this in just a moment. Your midwife will closely assess the wound and ensure there's no excess bleeding, oozing or unexpected smell coming from the wound site. I know this doesn't sound very pleasant, but please don't feel embarrassed; we've seen and smelt it all before and will do again and again after you.

It's normal to bleed after birth for up to a few weeks. Your placental wound site (the size of a dinner plate) needs to heal and the lining of your womb sheds. Some women are quite surprised at how heavy the bleeding is after birth and are alarmed by clots lost. You do need to let your midwife know if you're passing clots, but this is very common and usually nothing to worry about. Your midwife will assess any clots and be looking for placental tissue, so don't be surprised if they're having a rummage around in your blood clot. It may look odd, but we want to ensure there's no tissue left inside your uterus.

Tip: If you have any concerns over your blood loss, keep whatever is on your pad for us to have a look at! It's much easier for us to see rather than hear about.

Assessment and repair of any wounds

Between 85 and 90 per cent of first-time mums who give birth vaginally will have some form of perineal wound following childbirth. Of these, 70 per cent will require suturing after birth. If you have had a tear, remember just how common it is, even if women don't talk about it or you were not forewarned. Lots of mums tell me they had no idea about tearing and the process of suturing or wound healing. Part of what I campaign for, and have been for a while, is better education for women in general but especially in relation to the postnatal period. There are hundreds of thousands of (self-proclaimed) experts handing out birth preparation advice on every forum going, but there's not enough about what happens *after* birth. Therefore, when women have babies there are many surprises and taboos – tearing being one of the top ones.

Some mums have asked me how common tearing is because no one ever told them about it and they really thought they were among the few to sustain a tear to their perineum (the skin between the vagina and anus). The reason tearing is not discussed prior to birth is likely due to concerns over scaring mums, but withholding information can be more damaging in the long run. There are many ways to have difficult conversations with pregnant women that empower them and leave them feeling informed rather than scared.

There are very small and simple things that you can do to prevent perineal trauma, such as the choice of your place of birth (research shows that mums who give birth in a midwifery-led unit or at home have significantly reduced chances of perineal trauma). Birthing position and hydration of tissues are also important, both externally – such as with water immersion – and internally via drinking water prior to and during labour. Sometimes, no matter what you do to prevent a tear, it may still occur. But many mums don't know they have torn until midwives or doctors have a look and diagnose the type or grade of tear after birth. Please don't blame yourself.

It had been 150 years since a midwife invented a tool especially for perineal repair (stitches, also known as sutures, to repair tearing after birth). But an incredible Danish midwife, Malene Hegenberger, thought that was far too long and invented a device called the Hegenberger Retractor – the first and only device in the world designed by a midwife for perineal repair. It improves visibility for midwives and doctors while stitching and reduces pain for women undergoing the procedure. Malene is a true expert when it comes to suturing and has been a midwife for more than 22 years. I thought it would be good for her to share some of her advice around this topic too:

> 'Please speak up if pain relief is not working properly, and if the place you gave birth has gas and air you can supplement the local anaesthesia with this too. Just make sure you're still okay to hold the baby if they are with you or let someone else take over. If a tear has been stitched it is normal to have perineal pain for three to five days, but it is important that you feel a slow improvement. **If the pain continues or increases**, you need to be checked by a midwife or a doctor. I would recommend that you have a look at home with a mirror – it almost always feels different to how it looks.'

> Malene Hegenberger, midwife

As Malene says, it's common to have perineal pain for up to five days after having stitches, but thereafter the pain should be slowly but surely improving (see page 14 for tips on managing pain). If, however, the pain persists or worsens this is a very clear warning sign and possibly indicates infection or the need to reassess the suturing. Unfortunately, the wound will need to be reassessed as soon as possible. Early-onset infection is quite common and will usually need medicating with antibiotics. To prevent this, and also help manage infection, after having a shower wait a little before putting on underwear and maternity pads. Airflow helps to dry out your skin and therefore aids healing. It may not feel or look like it now, but you *will* heal; the vagina has a wonderful blood supply and tends to heal beautifully given the right environment.

YOUR BLADDER

During pregnancy, your organs become displaced to accommodate your growing baby. Your bladder is affected by the weight of your growing uterus, alongside hormones, and causes you to feel the urge to pee little and often. The usual wee window is between two and a half and four hours in a non-pregnant woman, although this will vary depending on how much you're drinking. Your bladder may have become used to more frequent urination. That's why it is important to consider retraining your bladder after birth and to remember that window, not immediately but as the weeks go by.

When it comes to passing urine after a vaginal birth, lots of mums report a stinging sensation if they have a wound or grazes (see page 14 for managing this). Your perineum can also be sore and swollen, and it may feel weird – almost like your perineum doesn't belong to you. This is quite common and usually resolves itself quickly. If ever you've got any concerns over the healing of your perineum or what it looks like, then, once again, talk to your midwife or ask for an assessment.

Postpartum urinary retention (PUR) is common in varying degrees and often means you can't wee within six hours of giving birth and, if you do, you may only wee a tiny amount. PUR is poorly researched and understood, but most often occurs if it's your first baby, you've had an epidural or spinal anaesthesia, you had a long labour or assisted birth, you had a tear or needed stitches, or you had a UTI or previous experiences of bladder problems. For this reason, your first urination post birth should be measured by your midwife. This is really important so please remind your midwife if you feel the need to go but they have not provided you with a jug. If you required a catheter during your labour or birth, then your midwife will usually request to measure at least your first three urines. There may be need to measure more should you not pass enough urine within these. PUR usually resolves itself within a few days, but please speak to your midwife about any symptoms you experience.

CATHETER CHAT

~~~

If you've had an epidural, spinal or general anaesthetic you would have had a catheter sited – this is a thin clear tube that's inserted via the urethra and remains in the bladder, draining your urine during the time you're less mobile and unable to take yourself off to the loo.

The catheter will need to come out after you've had your baby, and as mentioned previously, your midwives will assess your urine output to make sure you're emptying your bladder properly and look out for any signs of infection. Simply put, anything that goes into your body has the opportunity to cause infection, especially around that area. In case you're wondering, catheter removal isn't usually painful but may cause a slightly uncomfortable sensation. Usually after a C-section or an epidural, you may find that your first few wees feel odd or even uncomfortable. This will slowly improve and you'll feel more connected to your body. Infection, also known as a urinary tract infection (UTI), is more common after having a catheter. Symptoms of UTIs include:

- a temperature above 37.5°C
- dark or discoloured urine
- pain or stinging when passing urine
- feeling unwell
- feeling cold and shivery

The moment you start to feel any burning or stinging, try to flush out any potential infection that is brewing by drinking lots of water. If you are diagnosed with a UTI, you will likely need antibiotics, but your doctor will recommend and prescribe these. If you ever need antibiotics and are breastfeeding, always remind the prescribing clinician of this, just to make sure you take antibiotics that are safe for feeding.

POSTPARTUM POOING

~~~

Your bowels are also affected by the pressure and weight of your baby. Add to that the fact that increasing amounts of progesterone slow down bowel movement and cause constipation. Thanks again, pregnancy hormones! Your body needs to readjust, so your midwife will make sure your bladder and bowels are functioning well. They will ask you about your urine output and whether or not you have had a poo; this is usually disguised as, 'Have you opened your bowels yet?' There's honestly no need to feel embarrassed about being honest and saying you've had a poo. I know it's not the usual topic you'd discuss with someone you don't know well, but midwives just want to ensure your bowels are functioning as they should: pooing is part of human health.

Lots of mums are terrified to poo after sustaining any trauma, but especially if they needed stitches. This is a logical fear, but you won't damage your stitches. Malene Hegenberger advises:

'When going to have a bowel motion (poo), many women are afraid the stitches will break if they have to push. This is not the case. To help ease your worries you can use a clean hygiene pad and hold it gently against your perineum. In this way you gain control, and it feels easier to have a bowel motion. If you had a complex tear, seek out Facebook groups or organisations that support women through the healing process.'

Malene Hegenberger, midwife

Your first postpartum poo will generally be around a day or two after you have had your baby. Sometimes, though, medication or analgesia can cause a slight delay, especially opioid-based painkillers. Some mums report constipation too. This can be caused by the psychological concern over pooing and subconsciously holding on, reduced mobility or dehydration. Constipation is usually defined as having fewer than three poos per week. On the flip side, it's unlikely you have heard about leaking of poo (faecal incontinence) after birth, but it can happen, most commonly following an assisted birth or significant trauma to the perineum. Pressure and stress can injure your anal sphincter, leading to weakened control or temporary nerve/muscle damage. Please do not be embarrassed to speak to your midwife or doctor if this does happen. In most cases, with the right intervention and care, you will strengthen and regain control over this area. There are specialist teams of doctors and midwives that are able to help you retrain your bowels and assess your bowel function. After healing (and at least six weeks postpartum), you can also integrate some yoga practices, including Ashwini Mudra, which can help to strengthen the anus and pelvic floor together.

YOUR LEGS

You will be checked for any signs of blood clots in your calves, also known as DVT (deep vein thrombosis). If you're at an increased risk of DVT, you may be prescribed medication to take, which is usually a very small self-administered injection. Don't worry, you'll be taught how to do this at home. The medication thins your blood and therefore prevents clotting. Blood clots have become increasingly common over the years for a variety of reasons, including changes in human lifestyle. Calf pain, such as burning or stinging, along with isolated redness, one calf notably bigger than the other or severe breathlessness are symptoms you need to report *immediately* and have investigated.

Tip: While we're talking about legs, it is a good idea to get movement back into the body as soon as possible. Work within your restrictions and pain threshold. Movement does not even need to be walking; it can be circling your ankles while seated or in bed, or doing pelvic floor exercises, deep belly breathing which activates the transabdominal muscles, or head and neck stretches – any movement or stretching is positive.

HOW TO MANAGE PERINEAL PAIN

In the days after birth, many women get into the shower to wee because it eases the pain around external genitalia, and there is no problem doing that. Other women pour warm water from a jug over their vulva while weeing. This is also a very good way to ease pain and keep the area clean.

Lying on your side while breastfeeding will increase the venous blood flow from the legs through the pelvis towards your heart and decrease the pressure on your perineum and pelvic floor. In short, this helps with pain and healing, and may also have a calming effect.

Using cool pads (such as the type you can now buy that have inbuilt cooling gels) at home could ease the discomfort as well – just make sure you do not place any ice directly on your skin. This can cause more harm or even an ice burn . . . ouch!

With anything you experience, but especially infection, if we catch it early enough it shouldn't affect healing too much. If we don't, your healing can take significantly longer, increase your pain, or, worst-case scenario, you can become really unwell and need to be admitted into hospital. For that reason, I often recommend that mums take a look at any stitches and assess how well they're healing. Self-assessing can give you more control and you'll be able to report if things don't look or feel right. That said, it's really not for everyone and some mums are far too scared to look, so please do not push yourself to do anything that makes you feel uncomfortable. Remember, you can always ask your midwife or GP to have a look and assess your wound.

VISITORS

While we're on the subject of pain, visitors are either very welcome, a bit inconvenient, or outstay their welcome. The latter two are fairly common when I talk to new parents.

As exciting as it is for your loved ones to meet your baby, after birth you enter into a recovery process and anyone who is around you at that crucial time needs to be there for *you* and respect your needs. Eager friends and family mean well, but can make it awkward for parents to ask for space or set boundaries.

If this has happened to you and you feel like you can't say no, try to remember how precious these early hours, days and weeks are. You won't get this time back. You're not being rude or selfish if you don't want that time to be interrupted by lots of different people, and the more you strive to be upfront (to the people pleasers reading this – this is an important one for you), the happier you'll be in parenthood – but probably in general too. It can be liberating to be honest about what you want and parenthood is such a great place to start. You'll often need to try to stay true to yourself when your boundaries are challenged and care less about what other people think. Your needs deserve to be respected by you and the people around you. If you really can't say no then still try to set your boundary, such as: 'I'm really tired today and need to rest after lunch so could you visit from 10am to 11am?' That way you aren't left sitting there praying for them to leave and have made it clear the visit is on your terms. I know this sounds rather strict, but I really want to make sure your needs are protected – they're so important.

'Remember, you can change your mind. You might think when you're pregnant, "I want everyone to come and see me," and then you might have a really difficult birth or things might be trickier than you thought so you decide, "Actually, I don't want anyone to come. I just need to get some sleep and don't want to tidy the house." If you have a partner, get them to be the one to relay your wishes to everyone. Don't feel guilty – people can come and meet the baby at any point.'

Laura Smith, specialist community public health nurse (health visitor)
Ebonie Chandraraj, specialist community public health nurse (health visitor) @gentlehealthvisitors

If/when you have visitors remind them to bring you something or do something helpful during their visit. It's funny because I wrote about this in my first book and advise mums a lot on Instagram about setting the standards for visitors. So when I had Georgie and it was my turn, my visitors were very helpful! They brought me food, made me tea and really helped around the house. I do think that's because they knew what I wanted and expected. Sometimes it's just a case of letting people know how to help you. For anyone reading this and thinking, 'There's no way I can be so upfront,' remember you can still set gentle boundaries and frame things in a softer way while making sure their company supports you. For example, you could send a text ahead of their visit saying, 'I'm still very much recovering from the birth – it was exhausting! Would you mind . . . ?' (finish with whatever you feel most comfortable with).

VISITOR HELP LIST

Some practical ways your friends and family can lend a hand. They can:

- Top up your fridge/cupboards with essentials like eggs, bread, beans, etc.
- Bring a cooked meal.
- Help with organisation, such as putting any baby gifts that aren't for immediate use out of the way in a safe place/baby's room.
- Load/empty the dishwasher – if you have one – or do the washing-up.
- Find local support groups or classes, such as baby massage.
- Perform any other task you aren't able or don't want to do.

Overall, growing a human and giving birth is *a lot*. Give yourself time. The first 48 hours are about processing the birth, asking all the questions you need to and, of course, meeting your baby. Your care providers will be ensuring you are well clinically. As we've seen above, there are lots of observations and considerations. Always report any concerns and feel free to ask for second opinions if needed.

Birth experiences

YOUR BIRTH EXPERIENCE can leave you feeling a wide range of emotions that you flit between, so I want to dedicate some time to addressing those emotions here. The vast majority of these fluctuating emotions are normal and they usually pass or settle.

That said, some mums may need additional support or professional help to manage their thoughts, feelings and emotions after birth. We'll talk more about this on page 28.

Preventing birth trauma from occurring is a logical place to start, and is one of the many reasons I wrote my first book and created my online antenatal, birth preparation and postnatal courses, which you'll find on my website, www.themodernmidwife.com. But if you are struggling with your thoughts and feelings about birth, it's important to address this emotional response with the attention and respect it deserves. Let's move on to talk about that now.

HONESTY BOX

I gave birth in a birth pool in my living room and we have photos of those moments which I am so grateful for. I knew what to expect. Having seen so many women give birth in my time as a midwife, I naively thought I would have the ability to purposefully capture this moment in my mind. In reality I still can't clearly remember how I really felt – no matter how hard I try. I remember telling my midwives not to touch me or Georgie as her head was crowning. The stretching sensation was too overwhelming. She was born into my hands and I lifted her up out of the water myself. **It was the most empowering moment of my life.** The midwife in me couldn't help inspecting her as I normally would at work. I checked her heart rate and was calculating her APGAR score as she took her first breath. (The APGAR is a score out of 10 that's calculated at 1, 5 and 10 minutes after birth by assessing the baby's colour, heart rate, breathing, tone and grimace/reflexes.)

I decided to have a physiological third stage, so no uterotonic drugs or injections to deliver my placenta. It took a little bit of time to make an appearance so I used a midwife's old trick: had a wee and blew into an empty water bottle. Suddenly I felt pressure and delivered my placenta on the loo – in classic midwife style, shouting, 'Placenta out, minimal blood loss – what time is it please? There's no clock in here.'

A 'STRAIGHTFORWARD' PREGNANCY AND BIRTH

I have spoken to hundreds of women who have told me they don't think their feelings about their birth are justified, because, on paper, they had a 'straight-forward' birth. And they have been told that by almost everyone they have spoken to.

If you take anything from this section, take this: **there is no such thing as a straightforward pregnancy and birth**. You may have an amazing, empow-ering, fulfilling or even pleasurable experience, but growing a human, pushing them out of your vagina or having major abdominal surgery is never straight-forward. No matter what, we must respect how becoming a mother impacts women on both a physical and emotional level. Whether you had medical complications during pregnancy or birth or not, many women will still find it difficult, complicated, scary or shocking, and those feelings are justified. You do not need to feel ashamed of them. Instead, it is important to address and process them. I cannot stress this enough: **everything you feel is valid**, even if your birth was a positive experience.

The more we recognise, as a society, that having a healthy baby is totally inde-pendent from birth *experience*, the better we will become at really caring for mothers and acknowledging what women go through to bring another person into this world. You can have a healthy baby and be very grateful for that, but still feel sad about your birth experience or resent what you had to go through to become a mother. The two things are not mutually exclusive.

'We tried for over a year to get pregnant. Every time I got my period I felt so deflated. Finally we went for fertility treatment. I had to take a lot of drugs but we were ecstatic to become pregnant first time round. I found pregnancy difficult. There was so much advice out there – I googled everything and stressed a lot about how the baby was doing all the time. I had irregular bleeding throughout, borderline raised blood pressure, some concerns over the baby's growth. Our scans made me feel anxious every time: what if I were walking into bad news? How would I cope? When I got to 39 weeks, I decided to take the induction on offer. I had a bad experience to say the least; it took days and ended in an emergency C-section. When my baby was finally born, I felt numb – that's the only word I can use to describe it. The whole journey had been such hard work. I'm grateful to have been able to have a baby; it was just a real emotional rollercoaster and physical fight that no one really seemed to acknowledge. People expected me to be happy and I felt as though I would be seen as ungrateful if I was honest. So I lied a lot – to a lot of people – and put on a fake smile. Perhaps that contributed to my postnatal depression.'

Anonymous, mum of one

You may have had a birth plan and done absolutely everything in your power to achieve it, yet nothing went according to the plan. Birth is unpredictable. Mourning the birth you set yourself up for, worked so hard towards and dreamt about is totally acceptable, mama. In any other life situation, if you work towards something and it doesn't pan out, you allow yourself to feel disappointed. You have the right to feel the same way about your birth if it didn't go to plan.

It's also very important to note here that deviations from your birth plan are not your fault. Sadly, mums can feel as though they failed themselves or their baby if they require intervention or change their mind. There's a narrative floating around that says that, 'If you just try hard enough, if you refuse everything you're offered, if you breathe how you've been taught to, you'll get the birth you want.' This is simply not true and it's a dangerous narrative for mums to be led to believe. Mums *do* have control over many aspects of their birth, breathing *does* help and, where safe/appropriate, being in your home environment will support physiology; after all the body is designed to give birth, and when at home we give the body the opportunity to perform optimally. In a clinical setting the natural workings of a woman's body (which have been evolving for millions of years and best work in an environment mum feels most safe in) may be disturbed. This is because she's in a foreign environment, one that is often associated with illness, and she's cared for mostly by strangers. This can make her feel uneasy and therefore less likely to tune in to her primal brain, which is required for birth and the necessary release of birth hormones such as oxytocin. Homebirth is also proven to be safer than hospital for women with low-risk pregnancies. A home or midwifery-led setting often leads to less intervention and a more positive experience, with mum feeling in control and empowered as opposed to feeling like things are being done to her by the medical professionals around her. **But** that is not true for all mums, and women are entitled to change course, seek medical support or more analgesia, and must not be blamed for any deviation from a birth plan.

Birth is not about trying; it's about doing and it's unpredictable. I hope this section will help you find the confidence to have conversations and seek any support you deserve in order to better understand and process your birth and go easy on yourself for choosing a different option at the time.

A COMPLICATED OR TRAUMATIC BIRTH

Sadly, some births lead to serious complications, such as significant blood loss, uterine rupture or sepsis (overwhelming infection). This can be for a variety of reasons, and complications may be anticipated, or labour may take a sudden, unexpected turn.

Sometimes women feel anger towards their birth team or healthcare professionals if they feel like they took over, didn't listen, badly managed the situation or, worse, coerced them into agreeing to interventions they didn't want. A traumatic birth can also leave you *very* fearful of birth and therefore of having another baby – in case it happens again. I can't tell you how many mums have come to me, in my professional work environment and online, saying, 'I had a traumatic birth and am terrified of having another baby. If I do, can I have a planned C-section?' If you're wondering the same thing, the answer is yes. You can absolutely have an elective C-section, but it is important to explore all your options, talk to a range of birth workers and experts, and create a birth plan that covers everything you need in order to have a positive experience. An elective C-section may not be the only answer. After exploring options and having conversations with experts, you may find there's something else you need in order to achieve the birth experience you want. Although nothing can change the difficult experience of birth you have had, learning about how to prevent this from happening again and having a positive birth following trauma can really help you heal.

On the flip side, I also commonly receive messages such as: 'I had a terrible experience with my first baby. I hate hospitals and I just want to have my baby in the comfort of my own home. Can I have a home birth?' The answer to this is simply you can do whatever you want to do. In the UK we do not have laws to stop women giving birth wherever they wish to. However, in some cases there are certain medical conditions or complications that make hospital birth a safer option. There are many variables associated with birth so I can't give advice on safety for all, but what I can say is, speak to a range of professionals, ask for evidence-based statistics and absolute risk, consider the benefits of a home birth (because there are many), and know your birth rights.

You can overcome trauma and you can go on to have the positive birth experience that you deserve. You just need the right support and professionals who know how to help *you*. The single most important factor for mums who have a traumatic or complicated birth is that they **have a debrief or professional counselling/therapy** when appropriate. If you do opt for this or are considering it, please do not feel any shame in seeking support or feel as though it was you who failed. I can promise you, no one fails at labour or birth and I am deeply sorry that you walked away from birth with trauma. All of your emotions are valid and you will be able to overcome them with time and support. You're doing amazing at learning how to deal and cope with your trauma.

'At least baby is fine' is not an appropriate answer to your trauma, so it's important you do not adopt that as a viable solution to addressing and healing from birth trauma or PTSD. If you feel you need support for your birth experience you can:

- Ask for a debrief from the specialist team at the hospital where you gave birth.
- Check out the Birth Trauma Association, Make Birth Better or PANDAS Foundation (see page 241 onwards).
- Speak to your health visitor or GP.

The charity Birth Trauma Association estimates that 30,000 women suffer with birth trauma in the UK alone, every year. It can be hard to identify symptoms while you're experiencing them, and some mums pass these symptoms off as 'normal', so let's run through some of them now. They could include:

- flashbacks
- feeling irritable
- panic attacks
- numbness
- nightmares
- anxiety
- insomnia

Women often describe their trauma as 'living inside the birth experience' and find it difficult to escape their memories of it.

My doula, Kat King, has been a qualified yoga teacher for over a decade and specialises in pregnancy and birth, and has a real interest in healing and recovery after birth. She runs a programme called the 'Three-Step Rewind', which aims to help mums manage their emotions and repetitive thoughts about their birth. I asked her to share some more detail:

'The "Three-Step Rewind" was originally created by the originators of NLP [neuro-linguistic programming] and was known as "visual kinaesthetic dissociation" or phobia cure. It is a very clear and simple NLP/pattern technique that can help with feelings towards birth. It is a gentle but very effective process for de-traumatising people.

'The process is usually done over two to three sessions. You would be in a safe space to be guided through a pattern of suggestion which helps you to detach from the difficult heavy emotions attached to the memory of the birth. Your memory is still there; however, the aim, once completing the Three-Step Rewind, is that the memory will not evoke any negative association with the birth.

'Contact Birthing Awareness for a practitioner in your area [see page 241].'

Kat King, doula and yoga teacher, Loveuyoga

Kat has kindly supplied a few prompts to help you get started on your own:

THINGS TO JOURNAL ABOUT AT HOME

- What do you want instead of what you have now?
- When, where and how do you want to have the feelings you say you want?
- What are you going to begin doing now to get what you want?
- How will you know when you have got it?

A SHORT LABOUR

Lots of mums who have a very quick birth tell me their well-meaning friends or family often tell them how lucky they are, but 'luck' is not always something they can relate to. In fact, women who have very quick births can be in shock for a while or even traumatised. You have probably heard someone refer to an event that unfolded quickly by saying, 'It all happened so fast – I didn't have time to think.' When you don't have time to think, your brain needs to do the thinking afterwards in order to process the event and deal with the stress caused.

Just because you had a quick birth does not mean you escaped any of the physical discomfort or emotional upheaval of birth. Some mums do have very positive experiences with quick births, but not always. Intense sensations may have suddenly taken over your body, not giving you enough time to come to terms with what was actually happening in those moments. Perhaps you didn't have time to implement the tools you had learnt during pregnancy, like hypnobirthing. Or maybe you wanted stronger pain relief, such as an epidural, but were unable to because you were so close to giving birth. You may not have felt prepared for birth or motherhood, and suddenly it was happening and there was no going back. On occasions this can even lead to feelings of disconnect with your own body and your baby. It takes time to sink in. It's therefore completely normal to have lots of questions or to feel as though you need to keep talking about it in order to digest your birth experience.

If you can relate to this experience, it's a good idea to ask every question you have and tell your birth story as many times as you need to in order to help you process it. This is an important part of your emotional healing after birth. Psychologists understand the power of talking about an experience. So if you do feel like talking about it, let it all out and support your brain to process your experience.

Tip: Try to avoid taking note of other people's perception of *your* experience, especially if it is based on their experience – that's just not relevant to you. Acknowledge and validate your own emotions rather than falling into the trap of comparing your birth experience with someone else's.

HONESTY BOX

I have explained many times throughout my career that 'around 80 per cent of first-time mums go overdue'. So when I was given a due date during my first pregnancy, I hedged my bets and picked a date one week after my due date, often referring to that as my due date. Yet at 37 weeks plus two days I started getting some backache and period pains in the morning, had a show (lost my mucus plug) in the afternoon, and by 9pm I was in active labour – refusing to let my partner, Andy, call anyone. As odd as it may sound, and as much as I tell expectant mums 'there's a five-week window of normality from 37 to 42 weeks', I just could not accept that I was in labour and 'it' was really happening. We had another four weeks to go in my head. So when Georgie was born quite quickly at home, I was in shock for many months.

Our birth was a very positive experience. I felt so strong and supported, but one thing I didn't feel was ready. I know that may seem strange for someone with my experience and understanding, but it's the truth. I remember my due date arriving and looking at Georgie and thinking, 'How on earth are you here already? What has happened? I have actually had a baby.' One thing that really helped me come to terms with the shock was telling my birth story. Whenever I had the opportunity I would talk about it – and still do now.

A LONG LABOUR

Conversely, I have also spoken to and cared for lots of mums who have had long labours – really long labours. So long that by the time they have given birth they're utterly exhausted, and perhaps even delirious from days with minimal sleep or food. It's so sad to see a new mum in this way, often as a result of women not being listened to or birth being over-medicalised – which is where there is too much intervention during birth, hindering a woman's natural female physiology and making her feel inadequate. Often women feel as though their bodies have failed them, but it is sometimes possible that the guidelines failed them more than anything else. I don't want to portray birth or obstetrics in a bad light, but I think it's important to shed light on the reality women sometimes face. And, if the above is similar to your experience, I want to provide you with some much-needed support and recognition.

'I planned a home birth but had to be transferred into hospital because there was meconium in my waters. After a few hours of being there, I knew I wasn't going to give birth vaginally. I asked for a C-section so many times and was told it's better to keep going – have the drip and see what happens. My body was pushed to its limits for hours on end before going for an emergency C-section. I was right; at the section they said she would have never been born vaginally due to her position. I felt the team in hospital didn't listen to me and my intuition. Such a shame and could have saved me many hours of discomfort leading to exhaustion by the time she was born.'

Robyn, mum of one

A long labour can affect you for months after birth and it may feel like you struggle to overcome the exhaustion. Yet it's hardly ever spoken about (we cover postnatal depletion in more detail on page 28). In fact, some health professionals won't consider you to be in labour until you are 4cm dilated and having regular contractions, dismissing your claim to have been in labour for days. Not only can this be frustrating, it can also make you doubt yourself and your ability to judge what is happening to *your* body. Clinicians/birth workers need parameters and guidelines to work within so that they are able to provide standardised care and ensure that mums who are likely to give birth very soon are prioritised for one-to-one care. With staff shortages becoming a critical problem in maternity, it can be even harder to provide additional care outside of those guidelines. By no means am I saying this is acceptable – it is difficult for everyone. Most midwives wish they could provide more care or spend longer with mums in early labour. But my point here is that you are the expert when it comes to your body, and the only person on earth who really knows what you experienced is YOU.

Just because a labour has not yet qualified as being 'active' does not mean you're not experiencing contractions which may or may not take your breath away or prevent you from resting or going about your day. (That said, my advice to pregnant women remains the same: if you are planning a vaginal birth and have not had any complications, the best thing you can do when you start having contractions is *ignore* them until you can't ignore them anymore. Focusing on them, counting, messaging your WhatsApp group or getting yourself worked up will likely delay things. Sometimes, no matter what you do, some labours will be longer – this is usually due to the position of the baby in your pelvis and the descent of your baby and space.)

Many women go on to have a 'straightforward' vaginal birth after a long latent phase. Yet it was anything but straightforward for them because they had to endure many hours of feeling uncomfortable and potentially unheard, and are therefore left feeling irritable and fatigued. None of those outcomes are considered to be medical complications and can therefore be overlooked or not addressed. For the women who experience these feelings it is hard. Without processing or validating your experiences, negative emotions can fester or grow, and the thought of having another baby may lead to anxiety. But don't worry because it's never too early or too late to validate your experience.

According to researchers, a person who feels that their emotions are not wrong or inappropriate is more likely to have a solid sense of identity and worth and can manage emotions more effectively. Furthermore, emotional validation helps open the door to self-compassion. Feeling that our emotions are valid helps us avoid shame and self-blame, so we can respond to them with confidence. Nurturing, accepting and being self-compassionate are key to emotional recovery and mental wellbeing at any time, but especially after having a baby. If no one else is validating your feelings then it's important that you do. Check in on that self-chatter and make sure it's kind – whenever possible. I know it's not always easy and you can slip into talking down to yourself or giving yourself a good old dose of mum guilt, but observing your inner chatter can help you push it in a better direction. Take a few minutes throughout the postnatal period to breathe deeply and fully, and say to yourself, 'My feelings are valid. I give myself permission to feel this emotion.'

THE CONTEXT WE ARE TRYING TO BE MOTHERS IN

〜〜

You're allowed to complain about your baby and motherhood. Many mums feel they aren't allowed to say how they really feel. Yet if you were having difficulty with a colleague or a friend's behaviour, you'd feel it was okay to vent. With motherhood, many women feel as though they can't possibly vent about their child in the same way. They feel as though they are 'not allowed' to complain, as the squeaky-clean images we see in the media of new mothers don't make us feel safe in admitting we may sometimes find our responsibilities and our babies difficult. To the extent that, on some days, you may feel as though you just want to run away or check into a hotel with an already-made bed and clean sheets. And sleep or rest.

We can love our babies very much, but also find it extremely hard. Motherhood is full of contrasts, feelings of love and positivity alongside dark and challenging times, in a context where we may not feel all that well supported or understood. I promise you're not alone if you feel like this – these thoughts are common and it's okay to admit how you feel. The more we release, open up and are honest, hopefully, in time, the better we will be understood. You're doing great.

CARING FOR YOUR MENTAL HEALTH AFTER BIRTH

Some mums need professional support to help manage their thoughts and emotions after birth. If this is you, please know just how common this is. In the UK, up to 20 per cent of mums are diagnosed with postnatal depression (PND), and suicide remains the leading cause of death for mums in the perinatal period (during pregnancy and the year following birth). I strongly suspect the statistic on depression is higher, as sadly some mums won't feel able to report how they feel and therefore won't get a diagnosis.

PND isn't usually seen in mums until several days after birth and part of the diagnosis is looking at the length of time symptoms have been present. That said, if you feel as though you are becoming depressed, you feel low, have a change in appetite, are not enjoying things you usually would or have frightening thoughts about harming yourself or your baby, please do tell someone. I want you to know now that you won't have your baby taken away just because you have been honest about these thoughts. All healthcare professionals aim to keep a mother and baby together. Even in extreme cases of PND, mums and babies are almost always kept together. The intention of care providers is to support you to feel well again and keep you and your baby together.

The simplest way to know whether or not you need to speak to someone is if you get the thought 'I wonder if I have PND?' The fact that you think this is a possibility makes it likely you do need some level of support, and that's perfectly okay. It doesn't mean you're not coping or are any less of a mother than anyone else. It means you're dealing with the huge transition to motherhood, you're hormonal, sleep-deprived and perhaps have other factors impacting your adjustment. But, most importantly, it means that you know yourself and have identified that something isn't as it usually is.

Meeting your newborn

THE MOMENT YOU hold your baby for the first time may leave you with a vivid memory that you can relive, but for most mums, meeting their baby is a bit of a haze and difficult to remember clearly. As we've seen, birth can be overwhelming, even for mums who have a very positive experience.

EXPLORING YOUR BABY'S BEAUTIFUL BODY

The early hours after birth are often referred to as the 'hours of enchantment' by midwives as mums and babies meet and the process of falling in love begins. It can take longer than a few hours for this love to develop and flourish or it may happen right away. Exploring your whole baby takes time, and rightly so. Where possible, you don't want to rush this exploration. Many mums start by looking at their little face and all their tiny facial features, from their eyebrows to their lashes and their lips, and work your way down and around their body. Their little hands and fingernails are all unique to your beautiful baby. There's a lot to take in. I clearly remember a mum sitting up quickly in bed on the postnatal ward and saying, 'I can't believe it! I haven't seen her bum yet! Let me undress her!' The satisfaction after seeing the final part of her baby's body was a moment I won't forget. It stuck with me, how important that is, for parents to really see their baby and their baby's entire body.

A WHOLE NEW WORLD

Newborns are the closest we will come to a pure expression of our genetics. Their innate behaviour, alongside their ability to learn and willingness to communicate, is truly extraordinary. But let's not sugar-coat things – it may not feel extraordinary for you at 3am when you are exhausted, bleeding and have a baby crying for seemingly no apparent reason. On pages 117–126 there's a whole section specifically about crying, but, for the purpose of this section, the most common reason for your baby to cry within the first 48 hours is hunger or comfort and the need to be on you.

The early hours following birth are not just about bonding – this time is also about gentle adjustment to life on earth. Your baby has gone from the dark warmth of the womb, where noises are muffled and the constant, regular rhythm of your heartbeat is predictable and reassuring, to a bright, loud, comparatively chilly environment where there's no fluid on tap. It's all a bit overwhelming. Then, to top it off, they need to breathe independently and take over the work of the mighty placenta. Babies don't have the neurological capacity to understand what is happening, but they feel a huge change.

There's a lot you can do to support your baby through this period of adjustment and good old skin-to-skin contact ticks many of the boxes (see page 111). It's a bit of an outdated idea, that babies should be happy to sleep on their own in cots quietly. It is totally normal for newborns to protest against being apart from you and to get upset when they are placed in their cot. This can be exhausting for you, I know, so bear in mind that skin-to-skin does not have to be with you. It can be with any loving caregiver. It still keeps your baby lovely and warm, feeling safe and able to hear the familiar sound of a heartbeat.

YOUR NEWBORN'S REFLEXES

Newborns come into the world with some amazing reflexes that I can almost guarantee you'll soon spot! When a baby feels a loss of support or as though they are falling, the involuntary primitive response is to thrust their arms out wide and back in towards themselves. This is known as the Moro reflex. This reflex is thought to help the baby grip on to their mum if they were falling. The rooting reflex I find adorable, and involves head-bobbing as a way of searching for food. Newborns will also crawl to the breast at birth when left to their own devices. Here you'll see the rooting reflex at its finest! They are smelling and looking for the breast, while working their way to it using their arms and legs. There are many other reflexes, such as the sucking, grasp, tonic neck or stepping reflex, and these innate behaviours are incredible to watch – they remind me of how clever the human body and brain really are.

YOUR BABY'S EYESIGHT

At birth, the retina is very immature and photo receptors are inefficient, creating particularly blurred vision – it is about twice as poor as someone who is clinically blind. Colours are also muted for newborns. That's why it's a good idea to get up close to your baby. You may find you instinctively bring your baby close to your face and breathe them in or explore them at close proximity.

You may also notice your baby going cross-eyed and having trouble focusing. This is very normal and they will soon be able to focus better. That said, if you have any concerns over your baby's eye movement, always seek advice from your midwife or health visitor. Follow your instincts, but do know that the vast majority of the time this is quite normal for newborns.

THE IMPORTANCE OF SMELL

Your baby has a highly developed sense of smell and can recognise your scent – from birth. For babies, smell is critical for attachment because smells (or olfactory cues) are one of the main ways a baby recognises their mother and therefore safety. Their sense of smell appears to make up for what they lack in sight. The strength of a baby's sense of smell will never be found again in an adult; it is particularly impressive.

Ruth Feldman, Simms-Mann Professor of Developmental Social Neuroscience at the Interdisciplinary Center (IDC) Herzliya, Israel, wanted to find out more. Her team of researchers undertook a study to find out how the presence of a mother's scent impacted her baby while in the company of a stranger. In summary, when babies were able to smell their mum, they looked at the stranger more, smiled more, appeared to feel safer and showed more interest in the stranger. Whether mums were breastfeeding or not made no obvious difference to the results. Overall, babies appeared calmer in the presence of their mother's smell when autonomic response (involuntary physiologic processes like heart rate, blood pressure, respiration and digestion) was measured. There appeared to be a stress reduction but increase in alertness. These are important findings and something worth considering if your baby needs to be away from you at any time for any reason.

Smell is arguably the only sensory cue that can represent you when you're not there. This may be a powerful tool for you to use should you want or need to leave your baby, transmitting your comfort and safety through your scent, in your absence. Your baby may be able to bond with others and feel calmer if an element of you remains with them.

HONESTY BOX

After I had Georgie I didn't want to wear deodorant. She was born in August in the middle of a heatwave. We were advised to socially distance around that time because of the COVID-19 pandemic, so luckily it was mostly Andy who was exposed to my natural scent . . . My desire not to mask my bodily scent was an instinctive decision for me, bringing me to research how maternal scent impacts babies. The findings are powerful and I'm now glad I followed my instincts.

'I don't go out-out that much, but I had a run of hen dos and things planned with the girls. Every couple of weeks or so I was out on a Saturday night and home late. My youngest had slept through from a fairly young age. Her dad works late so she is used to hearing people come in late at night. But every single time I came in from a night out she would wake up. My husband says she sits up and looks around. She senses I am home. She's still breastfeeding and I wonder if it's the milk she can smell wafting through the front door.'

Michelle, mum of two

ADMISSION TO NEONATAL INTENSIVE CARE UNIT (NICU)

I really hope you were with your baby from birth for as long as you chose to be. Sadly, this is not always the case if babies need to go to special care. One of the most common reasons babies are admitted into NICU is because of prematurity. According to the World Health Organization (WHO), globally 15 million babies are born prematurely every year; 60 per cent of these births take place in Africa and South Asia. Around 1 in 13 babies are born prematurely in the UK. The separation can be agonising alongside the unknown. Questions abound around how long your baby will be in special care, exactly what they will need to help them remain stable, whether you will be able to hold them as much as you would like and how well they will feed. All of these concerns can exacerbate the enormity of motherhood and leave you in shock or survival mode. Remember, there are lots of professionals and specialists on hand to answer your questions so never be afraid to ask questions. There's no such thing as a silly question and a professional will never judge you for not knowing. Your questions are always valid.

Skin-to-skin as early and often as possible (see page 111), or 'kangaroo care' as it's often referred to, is particularly important for premature babies. There has been a lot of research into skin-to-skin and I have personally watched a tiny baby go from distressed to very calm, snuggling into their mum, during skin-to-skin contact. It is just incredible to watch as mums too are flooded with emotion and love. Remember the study above about smell and how babies calmed down when they could smell their mothers? It may be worth chatting to neonatal staff about how you can safely place an item that smells like you in with your baby. Some mums put little teddies down their tops for a few hours and then leave them in the incubator/cot with their baby. This is a lovely way of letting your little one know that Mummy is there.

For some parents it's not until their baby is discharged home that they start to process what happened and struggle with the emotional difficulties they faced. Resources to support you during this time and after can be found on pages 241–2.

TWINS

~~~~~~

The rate of twin births has rapidly increased over the past 20 years. Finding out you're pregnant with twins can be daunting. I have had many conversations with shocked and nervous parents about the concept of having two at once. There are various things you need to consider with twins, from equipment/products to feeding and additional support.

There's a lot of help available and some great charities. I love Twins Trust (see page 245) – their site is really easy to navigate and has so much information to help you during the first year. Some parents who have the budget for it opt for a twin specialist who offers home visits and help with getting set up. One thing most experts I have come across agree on is the importance of getting the twins into the same routine or schedule, as much as possible. This should be a routine that suits your whole family (see pages 144–7 for more on routine).

Feeding your baby

HOW YOU CHOOSE to feed your baby is personal and none of anyone else's business. There are many ways to feed your baby, from exclusive breast-feeding to bottle-feeding or expressing breast milk and combination feeding. Some mums start with one feeding method and switch to another, and that's perfectly okay. There's a lot of emotion and, sadly, mum-shaming attached to feeding, no matter what you do. Every mum has the right to make an informed decision and for that decision to be respected. Making informed choices may also involve requiring support as things unfold.

Actively seeking support is very different to being subjected to someone else's opinion regarding your personal situation. Many mums tell me they have been or are being pressurised around a certain feeding method. This pressure can be directed towards either bottle- or breastfeeding. Unless you ask for someone's advice or opinion, it's absolutely not acceptable for them to push any of their ideas, theories or opinions on what's best for you and your baby. If you ask for or welcome advice that's very different, and being supported or encouraged for the *right reasons* is what is important here. It's about time we respected a mother's choice and stopped telling women what to do with their bodies. We do not gear women up for the reality of breastfeeding in the UK. Instead, the media often shares a narrative that most women don't want to breastfeed, which means midwives are pushy about breastfeeding with moth-ers who want to bottle-feed, and we should leave these vulnerable women alone. This narrative is very rarely the case – as we'll go on to cover, the vast majority of mums do want to breastfeed; they just aren't given enough support and there's not enough funding for postnatal care.

Regardless of these political and cultural issues we face as new mothers, there's something really important I want you to know now: **however you decide to feed your baby, you can only do what is right for you at the time given your circumstances**. You do not need to feel guilty about how you choose to feed your baby. If you are feeling guilty, please talk about this to someone – bring it to light rather than trying to squash it down. Guilt is a very powerful emotion and it thrives on secrecy. You're not doing anything wrong at all. Don't let guilt trick you into thinking you are, mama. You're doing amazing, caring for your baby and your new self.

BREASTFEEDING AND REALISTIC EXPECTATIONS

In my first book I cover how to latch your baby on, avoid nipple pain and manage it if it does occur, plus the fascinating sci-fi-like facts about breast milk. It really is an incredible liquid packed with infection-fighting properties that are specifically designed for your baby, antibodies to many illnesses you've built immunity to; it provides optimal nutrition and reduces the chances of your baby developing conditions such as diabetes, asthma and heart disease, as well as SIDS (sudden infant death syndrome – see page 100 for more on this). These benefits are well publicised and it's more than likely you have heard about some if not all of them before. After all, NHS Digital reports that around 74 per cent of mums initiate breastfeeding. It would appear, then, that the majority of mums want to and plan to breastfeed. By eight weeks that drops to 45 per cent. At six months, around 1 per cent of mums are exclusively breastfeeding. This is a complex issue and I don't think there's an isolated reason for the huge gap between what mothers want or plan for and what happens six months down the line.

One thing I am certain about, and have seen many times with mums I have cared for, is the fact that the reality of breastfeeding is not discussed openly enough. I'm all for shouting about the benefits as long as this is backed with solid support and setting mums up with realistic expectations. The benefits mean nothing if you think your baby is starving because you haven't got enough milk, or you have bleeding nipples and are physically unable to put your baby to the breast. In those difficult situations, knowing the benefits may create nothing but a truckload of mum guilt when opting for formula. Let's not do that, mama – you don't need to carry any guilt ever; the motherhood load is more than enough to contend with – you deserve better. A huge part of what I do as a midwife is unpick unrealistic expectations and myths surrounding breastfeeding, so I would like to offer you some 'real talk' on the subject. As mentioned, there are different ways to feed your baby. First, we will focus on exclusive breastfeeding, which you may see midwives document in your notes as EBF – meaning your baby only has breast milk.

WINDING YOUR BABY

Some claim that breastfed babies do not need winding, but I think it's a good idea to wind all babies, no matter how they are fed. It's worth noting, though, that bottle-feeding can lead to babies sucking in more air.

There are different winding positions for you to try. I personally love winding a baby upright with their head just over my shoulder. This can feel lovely and secure as you support their bottom with one hand and wind with the other. Winding usually entails a circular-motion back rub with patting in between. You may also want to try sitting your baby on your knee, supporting their chin with one hand and using the other to wind.

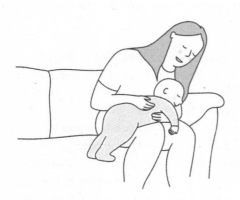
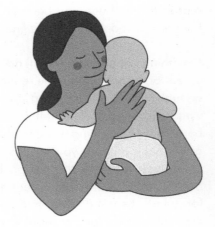

SETTING YOURSELF UP

Expectation, understanding newborn behaviour, supply and demand, good positioning, latch and attachment are key. But an integral part of all breast-feeding journeys is **support**. You need support from those around you, such as your partner, close family and friends, and experts. The UK has one of the lowest breastfeeding rates in the developed world – this is something that really needs to be addressed, but not by mothers. Women are not to be blamed or shamed for this; instead, we need to look at what we are doing differently to countries like Croatia, where there's a staggering 82.7 per cent breastfeeding rate. Breastfeeding difficulties are multifactorial, so every little thing can help, such as knowing where your local groups are, talking to a mum you know who has breastfed and asking her for advice or support, accessing the National Breastfeeding Helpline (see page 242 for the direct number and hours), following social media channels that offer solid support, and requesting some in-person guidance. This can be delivered either via the NHS, free of charge, or by seeking out a lactation consultant, which can be fairly pricey but fantastic if you have the budget for it.

RESPONSIVE BREASTFEEDING

Experts recommend that mums feed their babies responsively, but this is usu-ally a contradiction of what we are told or taught. We are taught that babies should follow a routine and fit into our lives, that we make a rod for our own back by cuddling babies too much and that babies are manipulating us. None of the above is true, nor does it support the responsive-feeding recommenda-tion. While introducing a gentle and adaptive routine may be helpful for some (and we'll cover this later, on pages 144–7), it often doesn't work within the early weeks of a baby's life.

In 2016 Unicef UK's Baby Friendly Initiative released an infosheet advising parents to feed their babies responsively: 'Responsive breastfeeding involves a mother responding to her baby's cues, as well as her own desire to feed her baby. Crucially, feeding responsively recognises that feeds are not just for nutrition, but also for love, comfort and reassurance between baby and mother.' Part of responsive feeding is getting to know your individual baby and what they want and need, rather than comparing or categorising them as 'good or bad'. There is no such thing as a naughty baby; they are just acting on instinct and are very honest about how they are feeling.

BREASTFEEDING TAKES TIME – MORE THAN YOU MAY HAVE THOUGHT

Usually breastfeeding takes time to get the hang of, but it also takes up a lot of your time to sit and feed or pump as you're the only person who's responsible for that. Sometimes mums find the amount of time required to feed, or to have to stop what they're doing to feed, difficult, leading to frustration or feelings of overwhelm. Many breastfeeding mums often refer to themselves as a 'milk machine' because their babies want feeding so regularly. Mums are generally very busy people and there's a misconception that maternity leave is a 'break'. Many mums have been shocked at the comments people have made about their time off, subtly insinuating they are sitting at home, not doing much. Being at home with a baby and breastfeeding that baby can be harder than any full-time 'job'. Raising the future is not an easy task, for the mind or body.

My point here is to ensure you are not misled by anyone else's expectations, or even your own of yourself. No one 'bounces back'; it takes time, energy and a lot of effort to sit down and feed your baby. If you're finding this hard, it's not because you're any less able than any other mum. You're finding it hard because it *is* hard and time-consuming. If you notice commitments or aspects of your life receiving less attention, it can be very hard to accept, whether that is missing out on a girls' night, the impact on your relationship, your skincare routine falling by the wayside, household maintenance being overlooked or another child or toddler not getting as much attention as you would like to give . . . the list goes on. It may seem like all you're doing is feeding and you don't have much time for anything else. If you do continue to breastfeed, remember the gaps between feeds do gradually get a little longer, giving you a bit more freedom.

Until these gaps get bigger and feeding is established, usually at around 6–8 weeks, life as a breastfeeding mum can be full-on. It's normal to find this intense and not the blissful, rosy picture you may have been led to expect by portrayals in the media.

All breastfeeding journeys differ, just like birth experiences. Some are shorter, some longer, some are more difficult and require more support or even inter-vention (such as tongue-tie release – see box opposite) and some are less complicated. Hardly any mum I speak to reports having an easy breastfeeding journey, though. Even if your baby latches on well, feeds like a dream and gains weight, sharing your body with another person is demanding, draining and can feel restrictive – depending on your lifestyle. Sometimes you will love every minute of a feed and feel truly fulfilled, connected, warm and fuzzy as the 'feel-good' hormone oxytocin floods your body. Other times you may feel 'touched out' and frankly want them to hurry up and finish the feed so you can move or complete whatever it was you were doing before you had to come to an abrupt stop. It's okay, mama – all the feels are normal and I'm going to keep reminding you of that. I'm very open about my own breastfeeding journey because I don't want you ever to feel as though your experience is abnormal or that you're a bad mum.

TONGUE-TIE

A tongue-tie (ankyloglossia) is where a line of tissue connecting the tongue to the bottom of the mouth is, most commonly, too short. The connecting tissue may also be too tight or too close to the gum. These very minor alterations of tissue can cause some difficulties, especially during breastfeeding, because they restrict the tongue's movement and therefore latch. Diagnosis is becoming more and more common – with entire clinics set up specially for tongue-tie release. You can't diagnose a tongue-tie by simply looking – a trained clinician will need to have a look and feel, observing how the tongue moves within the mouth. If you think your baby may have a tongue-tie, please speak to a healthcare professional as soon as possible. If you're unhappy with the advice, always feel free to seek a second opinion – you know your baby.

HONESTY BOX

Based on my experience as a midwife, I was fortunate to be able to ignore our culture's version of what's 'normal' for young babies and any questions about how 'good' my baby was. I set myself up with very realistic expectations ahead of starting out on my own breastfeeding journey with Georgie. I knew I'd be sitting there for hour upon hour, day and night, feeding intermittently, sometimes with very short gaps in between. I knew she would likely want to cluster-feed in the evenings (where babies feed with very short intervals) and that I'd be the main person responsible for making and providing her milk – I wanted to exclusively breastfeed for as long as possible. I therefore spent the first six weeks focusing on feeding and establishing that for the both of us. After helping so many mums, I felt confident in knowing when our latch wasn't right, so I'd take her off as many times as I needed to and re-latch her until it was optimal. I'd recommend you do the same to avoid sore nipples. Grinning and bearing it through pain during a feed is a temporary and unpleasant solution, usually causing long-term pain as well as impacting milk supply. Although the suction may feel strong or even uncomfortable, it should not be painful.

Even as an experienced midwife I still had to be really patient and persevere during the period of establishment. I still doubted myself at times too, especially through engorgement – my boob was way bigger than her little head, which resembled my childhood dolly. Even though I was equipped with experience and knowledge, I still found it really hard. Georgie was born a dinky 5lb 10oz and had a tiny little mouth, similar in size to a premature baby's. It was very tiring, helping her to latch and feed so frequently. On several occasions, I walked over to the formula in the supermarket and gazed at it for a few moments, wondering if I really wanted to continue. I fantasised about getting a full night's sleep and asking Andy to do the night feeds. I knew deep down that I didn't want to switch to formula-feeding and I did enjoy the feeds mostly, so I would walk away from the formula – usually towards the biscuit aisle. In tired times biscuits were something that did really help! As well as remembering that, once established and out of the first six weeks, I would be able to quickly pop her on the boob to settle her without fiddling around with the latch as much. I knew the boob would likely fix a lot – it's far more than nutrition. I also wouldn't need to worry about taking bottles out with me! I love travelling light so the thought of carrying anything else and being reliant on those extras put me off. My mum had breast cancer (she made a full recovery, thank goodness) so the knowledge that by breasfeeding I was reducing my risk of that and other cancers helped me through the tired times too. There will be slightly different motivations that help you when you're feeling a little fed up with all the feeding. Or perhaps not, and you'll decide to change course entirely, or to top with formula up and have a break – both are okay. You need to do what you feel is right at the time – guilt-free.

Tip: Your milk 'coming in' can be a real curveball as you think you have got the hang of breastfeeding, then it all changes because the shape of your nipple alters with the increased milk quantity and consistency. You therefore struggle with the latch. Positions that were working may not be effective anymore as it appears your baby is slipping off the breast. Ask for support here and try not to panic. You'll get them on the breast again. Sometimes reclining slightly to feed can help, or expressing some milk off to soften the breast may also enable a better latch. I have a full online postnatal course that covers breastfeeding and offers demonstrations – available on my website: www.themodernmidwife.com.

'I DON'T HAVE ENOUGH MILK'

Sometimes mums think or are told they don't have enough milk – it's up there as one of the most common misconceptions about breastfeeding. It is extremely rare for mums not to be able to produce enough milk. Although it's difficult to get an exact statistic on this, it is generally agreed among feeding experts that around 3–5 per cent of mums aren't able to make enough milk for their baby. The following can increase the chance of this happening:

- a major bleed after birth – usually more than 1.5 litres
- any previous injury, trauma or surgery to the breasts
- damage to your nerves or spinal cord
- very few or no changes at all to the breasts during pregnancy
- a history of radiation therapy
- conditions such as polycystic ovary syndrome (PCOS) or hyper/ hypothyroidism

If you have been diagnosed with or have a history of any of these and suspect you have low milk supply, please do speak to your doctor or midwife as there are things that can help if you want to start or continue breastfeeding.

ORAL THRUSH IN BABIES

Approximately 1 in 7 babies develop oral thrush, so it's common. Antibiotics given to either you (while breastfeeding) or your baby can increase the chances of thrush.

Some of the signs include:

- White spots or patches on the tongue, gums, roof of the mouth or the insides of their little cheeks. If you wipe these, they don't come off, unlike milk coating. You may also notice a white film on your baby's lips.
- Unsettled baby during a feed as thrush can cause soreness.
- Some babies also have nappy rash (known medically as 'napkin dermatitis') which tends not to clear up with the usual tips and tricks (see page 193). That's because it is caused by the same yeast infection.

During breastfeeding the infection has the opportunity to pass from their mouth to your nipples. This can be particularly painful, mama. I have seen it a few times. You'll need treatment from your GP if this does happen.

In most cases, oral thrush in babies will clear up on its own, but always seek medical advice if you are concerned, in pain, your baby isn't feeding well, or you think your baby needs treatment.

The concern over low milk supply is usually driven by the fact that newborns want to feed very regularly – probably far more than anticipated. Perceived insufficient milk supply is the major reason mums stop breastfeeding. Georgie fed almost hourly for weeks after birth. This was normal for her and, once we established breastfeeding, we got more time between feeds. I really think mums are misled by the advice to 'feed your baby every four hours'. I cringe now when I think that, as a junior midwife, that phrase was part of my discharge advice to new mums leaving the postnatal ward. After hearing about the four-hour window, mums may naturally think their baby will go around four hours between feeds, or perhaps assume they would need to wake the baby, reminding them to feed. But what tends to happen is that, when a baby wants feeding way more than every four hours, mums logically conclude they don't have enough milk and their baby must need a top-up with formula. When the baby then wants to cluster-feed (and no one explains this is part of newborn behaviour) it may confirm their conclusion that there's not enough milk, leading to mums topping up. By topping up, mums then usually miss a feed, creating the problem of low milk supply because the body makes less milk when there's less demand. Once begun, it can be hard work for a mum to break out of this cycle: you need to reverse the process and rebuild supply with very regular feeding/expressing/stimulating. Though topping up is some-times necessary, in my experience it is rarely needed for a clinical reason. If anyone advises you to top up with formula, I would encourage you to ensure that it really is *necessary*.

You can advocate for yourself and your baby in this situation by:

- Ensuring the person advising this is specifically trained to provide breastfeeding advice and support.
- Asking whether there are signs your baby is well fed. Generally these are: signs of a well-hydrated baby, weeing and pooing frequently with nice light-coloured urine, waking for feeds, alert, no signs of progressing jaundice and good muscle tone, to name a few.
- Asking about a plan to support you to continue to breastfeed if topping up is the safest option for your baby.

Tip: Increasing and protecting milk supply is absolutely key for breastfeeding mums, so if you do choose to top up, remember to **protect your supply** and continue to pump, hand-express and put your baby to the breast. If you skip a feed, your body gets the message 'We don't need as much milk as we thought, so dial down on the milk-making.'

DO BABIES REALLY LOSE WEIGHT?

It's very normal for newborns to lose weight after birth, especially if they're breastfed. This can cause a lot of concern for new parents and lead them to believe they need to top up with formula. Most hospitals and specialists will recommend that it's safe for newborn babies to lose up to 10 per cent of their birth weight. If a baby loses more than this, a top-up is often recommended, *but* it is important to consider and question these things before topping a baby up:

1. Were you given lots of fluid via your veins during birth? If so, ask whether this could have impacted your baby's birth weight.
2. What scales have been used? Are they the same? If not, is it possible to weigh the baby on the same make and model of scales?

3. Has the calculation been checked a few times to ensure it's correct? Sometimes weight loss can be miscalculated. Checking more than once helps to rule out errors. I have miscalculated in the past and rechecking has prevented a baby from being readmitted to hospital unnecessarily. This is an obvious but important point.

4. Is your baby displaying all other signs that they're well and not dehydrated (see page 49 for signs of dehydration)? For example, do they have good muscle tone and have regular wet and dirty nappies? Are they a healthy colour for their ethnicity? Do they not appear jaundiced? The symptoms of jaundice are lethargy, yellow-coloured eyes/skin and dark-coloured urine or fewer wet nappies than usual.

ALCOHOL AND BREASTFEEDING

It is a myth that you can't drink alcohol during your breastfeeding journey. It is certainly best to avoid alcohol in the first few months of your baby's life – because their liver is so immature and they feed very regularly – but once your baby has started to feed with longer intervals, if you would like a glass of wine or whatever tipple you prefer, you can safely time this with a feed. Alcohol can and does pass through to breast milk, so the timing and quantity of alcohol you consume are key to keeping your baby safe and avoiding them being exposed to alcohol. (We all metabolize at different rates, but the NHS advises waiting two hours after having a drink before feeding.)

Many mums want to and do drink while breastfeeding. I would therefore much rather cover how to do this safely than dish out outdated advice and deny mums some desired and well-deserved freedom.

As with your blood level of alcohol, the alcohol in your breast milk (if any has passed through at all) declines with time. Very small amounts of low-percentage alcohol, such as in a glass of Buck's fizz, are unlikely to reach your breast milk, so you don't need to be scared of enjoying a glass with your family during a special occasion, for example. It's important for you to enjoy yourself and not to feel isolated or excluded. We have a Boxing Day brunch, and home-made Buck's fizz was essential for me!

If you do like a drink, want more than a little tipple, or have a wild hen party to attend (enjoy!), remember that you can express ahead of time, store breast milk and give it to your baby in a bottle before a heavier drinking session. Bear in mind that your boobs might become uncomfortably full if you leave long gaps between feeds. It's best to express for both comfort and to keep up milk supply. Ideally, take a portable pump with you if you're away from home. You don't need to pump-and-dump to clear your milk of alcohol, though. The milk will only be clear once the level of alcohol falls in your body. So it's pointless getting as much out as possible in the hope of reducing levels.

A very important point if you are drinking is to consider the effects it has on you at the time – avoid being the main care provider for your baby. Try to make sure you drink plenty of water between the booze as this may help you to pace yourself and it reduces the effects of dehydration caused by alcohol. Hydration is really important while you're feeding and pumping. If you're having your first proper drink after having your baby, remember that your tolerance will be lower, meaning you will likely feel drunk much quicker. Lastly, speaking from experience, build in support for the following day. Hangovers with babies are never fun!

MAKING THE DECISION TO STOP BREASTFEEDING

I have looked after mums who, to support their mental health, have opted to give their baby formula. Your mental health is more important than almost anything. Motherhood is hard – and I am not talking about the general hardship of it now; some mums do need to be reassured that their baby's wakings are normal, or that their baby's behaviour is normal, and that they will eventually have longer gaps between feeds. But in other cases, where a mum is becoming mentally unstable and pushing herself into extremely dark places, a change of plan may be helpful. A mother may need to rest more in order to recover from the birth and feel well again, avoiding frequent night wakings. She may need someone else to feed her baby in order to sleep and rest. She may want to take stronger painkillers than recommended with breastfeeding. What's not okay is to expect a new mum, who's struggling with pain or mental health deterioration, to do it all.

Motherhood is full of occasions where you need to dig deep, find that last bit of patience, drag yourself up in the early hours of the morning to settle, support or calm your baby. You need strength and stamina. Sometimes something has to give to enable you to flourish in other areas that are important to you in your life. As a society and culture in the UK, we don't offer mums the support, care, attention and understanding they need. This applies even more so to breast-feeding mums; society does not protect breastfeeding mothers. As a midwife, I know how great breastfeeding is, but as a mum I know how hard it is too. I did become fed up with sharing my body for such a long period of my life. In total, it was 27 months of watching my caffeine intake, not drinking what I wanted, and not being able to apply products I wanted to use on myself. I just want you to know that you are the only person who can make the call regarding what you do with your body and whether you feel able to breastfeed.

We need to ensure you are well and do what you need to do to look after your-self. By looking after your mental health you're doing the best thing for your baby. It's very common for mums who stop breastfeeding earlier than planned to feel a wide range of emotions, including guilt and even grief. It really breaks my heart when I talk to mums and they are listing all the reasons why they stopped breastfeeding – as though they need to justify their decision, perhaps to me and to themselves, again. I usually respond with, 'I support whatever you chose and I hope you know you made the right choice at the time.' And the same goes for you, reading this. It's also okay to not want to breastfeed and to want more freedom. I have known mums who very candidly talk about why they don't want to breastfeed and prefer to have the opportunity to go out when they want, without worrying about feeding or pumping. Thinking like this does not make you a bad mum – you have the right to do what suits you. **There's no rule book you have to follow: you set the rules here**. It's your body, your choice.

SIGNS OF DEHYDRATION IN BABIES

Watch out for:

- a depressed fontanelle (that's the top of the baby's head and you may see it dipping inwards)
- dark-coloured urine
- reduced urine output
- lethargy

FORMULA-FEEDING

~~~~

As we know, in the UK 99 per cent of babies will receive some formula milk by six months, whether that's in combination with breast milk or on its own. Although breast milk will always come out on top when compared to formula nutritionally, bottle-feeding can be a beautiful bonding experience and release a surge of oxytocin, giving you all the warm fuzzy feelings too – especially if done skin-to-skin and while having eye contact. But don't worry, I'm not suggesting that every time you feed your baby you try to maintain eye contact throughout – that's just not realistic, especially if this is not your first baby and you have another child to look after. Keeping your baby close during a feed is really important for the two of you in those early days, though. It enables your baby to begin to recognise your face and it also activates areas of your brain associated with neurological synchrony (where your brain activity is mirrored, enhancing bonding and attachment). Babies also trust and feel safe with the person feeding them, no matter how they are being fed. Attachment is a crucial part of development, so by simply holding your baby close, having skin-to-skin contact or stroking their little body and talking to them, you're doing an incredible job of caring for your baby, keeping them safe and supporting their development.

When it comes to choosing a brand of formula for your baby, it's worth bearing in mind that all formula milk manufacturers have to follow very strict guidelines on ingredients, although some formulas are organic and others are not. It's best to do some research of your own into the various brands on offer, and bear in mind that some of the marketing around these formulas may be aimed simply at selling higher-priced ranges.

In terms of frequency of feeding, it's still recommended that you feed responsively, just like with breastfeeding (see pages 39–40). It's key to look for feeding cues as you would while breastfeeding too (see box over the page) and gently allow the baby to take the teat. Pacing feeds and watching your baby are also very important, so you know when they're full. Although you may see a little bit of formula left in the bottle, if a baby is full, always avoid encouraging them to finish the bottle. This can lead to overfeeding and may cause stress for both you and your baby. You should both be able to relax in the comfort of knowing there's no need to finish a bottle.

Tip: The muscles in the mouth and tongue used to suck from the breast are different to those used to suck a bottle. The milk usually flows a little easier from the bottle than the breast, especially within the first 48 hours. Therefore, babies can easily guzzle down milk and become very full, stretching their tiny marble-sized tummies. That's why it's important to pace a bottle-feed, and really observe the feed and how much your baby has taken. Stopping to assess this is a good idea and, while you do so, you can also take the opportunity to wind your baby and observe how the milk is settling, giving them a chance to feel full. You may also want to consider the range of teats available and whether there is a more suitable one that offers a slower milk flow.

FEEDING CUES

- Rooting around, head-bobbing or appearing to sniff the air – babies literally search for their food.
- Sucking anything in sight.
- Licking their lips, opening and closing their mouth.
- Bringing their hands to their mouth.
- Becoming restless.
- Rapid eye movement: they appear to be looking around for their food.
- Crying: this is the final feeding cue. Where possible, try to spot the earlier signs and feed your baby if you do.

Preparing the bottle

Following hygiene guidance on bottle-feeding and ensuring all feeding equipment is appropriately sterilised is very important. Babies have an immature immune system and are vulnerable to infection-causing bacteria. Preparing the bottle correctly is key to keeping your baby safe. When mixing formula, always use fresh water and measure it carefully according to the manufacturer's instructions on the label. Ensure that you are using fresh formula and discard any leftovers after a single feed. The timeframe for this will also be stated on the label. Always check the temperature of the formula on the inside of your wrist before giving it to your baby; it should feel warm or neutral, never hot.

Cleaning and sterilising

When cleaning bottles and teats, start by rinsing them with warm water and wiping away any leftover residue with a soft cloth or sponge. After this you have different options:

- Cold water sterilising using just tap water and a tablet.
- Boiling by placing them in a pot of water for ten minutes, making sure all feeding equipment is submerged – this will kill any bacteria or germs on them.
- Using an electric steriliser. Manufacturers will give guidelines on how long you can leave equipment in the steriliser before it needs to be sterilised again.

Caring for your newborn

THERE ARE A few common things that you need to be aware of when caring for your newborn in these very early days:

VERNIX CASEOSA (VC)

Aka 'birthday frosting', this wonderful stuff is a white, greasy biofilm that covers your baby during the last trimester. It's seen in variable amounts at birth, depending on their gestation at birth when the baby is born. For example, very overdue babies do not have much of it and premature babies can be covered in it. Vernix consists of water (80 per cent), proteins (10 per cent) and lipids (10 per cent), including barrier lipids such as ceramides, free fatty acids, phospholipids and cholesterol. That combo breakdown may not mean much to you, but it's the world's best moisturiser and has protected your baby's skin in the womb and is unique to humans.

Vernix has several important roles, including:

- Waterproofing: it protects the skin in utero from excessive water exposure during the development of the stratum corneum layer of the skin.
- Lubrication: it lubricates your baby's skin, helping your baby slide through the birth canal.
- Immunity: it provides a physical barrier to infection and contains lysozyme, lactoferrin and other components with antimicrobial activity. It also contains anti-inflammatory molecules, and has antioxidant and wound-healing properties.

Leaving the vernix on your baby's skin rather than removing it assists the development of the acid mantle – a really cool defence barrier on the surface of the skin that babies naturally build all by themselves when left to their own devices. The skin is the body's biggest organ and has many vital roles in promoting health. It's so important that we protect this natural process as much as possible. Leaving vernix to sink in and be absorbed is one thing you can do to support your baby's skin health. This also leads to significantly greater skin hydration and lower skin pH 24 hours after birth.

While we are on the topic of skin and optimising skin health, you may notice your baby starts to get dry skin that starts peeling, or they develop 'cradle cap'. This is a very normal part of the skin's changes and adaptations to life outside the womb. More often than not, skin peeling on the body doesn't need anything to support it and the skin will gradually peel off, leaving beautiful, healthy and intact skin underneath.

Cradle cap is often seen as patches of thicker scaly, white/grey skin on the head. If you are a scab picker – like me – as tempting as it may be to get a fingernail underneath and lift it off, avoid picking any dry skin. Picking can cause pain and damage the skin. Some suggest using a soft brush to lightly loosen it, then a shampoo. I do not advise this unless it's severe. Using shampoo isn't often necessary until your baby is over six months, and I believe in leaving the skin alone as much as possible for as long as possible. I didn't use shampoo on Georgie until she was over one – we just washed her hair with plain water in the bath.

CORD CARE

Newborns all have a cord 'stump' from their umbilicus (belly button) when the cord is cut. The cord then goes dark, shrivels up, dries out and, eventually, falls off. This usually falls off by the time you're discharged from your midwife around day 10–14. Some people like to keep it; others not. It is, of course, up to you, but I'll warn you – it can have a bit of a funky smell. Some cords can take a bit longer to fall off. I have heard of stubborn cords staying on for several weeks! Your midwife will monitor the shrivelling progress with you and look out for signs of infection.

The key cord-care tips are as follows:

1. Try to avoid handling it as this may increase the chances of infection.

2. Avoid washing it, so as not to disrupt the delicate natural flora – we have become obsessed with 'anti-bac' and washing, but washing newborns can cause more harm than good (see page 184).

3. When you change nappies, make sure you leave the cord outside of the nappy as contact with wee or poo may interfere with healing/drying. This does mean that some 'gunk' from the cord may be left on baby's clothes (if they are dressed right away) but it usually comes out in a hot wash. This is one reason I recommend white in the early days, as you can boil-wash that colour.

4. Once the cord falls off, there may be some minor bleeding, but if you have any concerns over your baby's belly button, bleeding, smell or anything else, please contact your midwife immediately.

NAPPY CHANGING

Changing your baby's nappy can be a daunting task, especially for parents who have never done it before. There's no need to feel awkward or embarrassed about this – if you haven't had a baby before or been around babies, why would you have changed one? There are no criteria you need to have met to become a parent, and no one is assessing your nappy-changing ability, so please don't worry.

Although you do, of course, need to be gentle, try not to focus too much on how delicate your baby appears. Babies are rather resilient and have either been pushed through the birth canal and had their entire body squeezed, or been handled out of your tummy by a doctor – perhaps with the assistance of some instruments, depending on their position. Holding their legs up out of the way isn't going to harm them, although they may scream like it is! It's always worth checking the surface they're lying on and aiming for it to be warm if they're naked, or putting something nice and comfy under them, but, even with these considerations, babies will often get very upset during a nappy change and being wiped. Something else that can reduce their irritability is using warm water and cotton wool in those very early days and transition to wipes once they're a little more used to being changed.

I'm sure you already know this, but when a little girl has pooed it's important to wipe from the front (vulva) to the back (anus) to avoid poo getting into the vagina or urethra (pee hole). Ensure you pass this on to whoever else is changing them too. Make sure you clean the vulva properly and avoid getting poo into the entrance of the vagina. This can be hard, so wiping gently around the area is best, rather than one central wipe down.

With little boys, be prepared for a wee as soon as that nappy comes off, as the cool air can stimulate them to pee. I once changed a little boy for a tired mum and had a cup of tea underneath the changing station; he peed right into my cuppa – charming! Ensure you keep your baby's penis covered or have something nearby to catch/direct the urine. You do not need to try to pull back their foreskin – just wipe the poo away from front (scrotum) to back (anus) and ensure the little folds of skin are nice and clean. You also need to ensure they are clean around the testicles.

MINI PERIOD

Baby girls also sometimes bleed a bit or have a white, cloudy discharge coming from the vagina. I have had many calls from worried parents about this. It's usually nothing to worry about and quite normal – this little bit of pink loss or discharge is caused by hormones passing from you to your baby before birth. That said, if your baby did not receive vitamin K, it's really important to report any bleeding immediately so they can be assessed appropriately.

While we are on the topic of the reproductive system, I must add an amazing fact here about newborn females: baby girls are born with all the eggs that they will ever have. For that reason, our cellular life as an egg began in the womb of our grandmother. A part of us lived in our grandmother's womb – for around five months. How incredible is that?

KEY POINTS

- You may experience many physical symptoms after birth as your body begins its journey through recovery.
- Report any concerns to your midwife or doctor and do not put up with pain. This may delay healing.

- Birth creates a permanent change, requires a significant amount of energy and leaves mums feeling a wide range of emotions. Ensure you protect the early hours as much as possible, with minimal intervention; keep lighting low and voices soft, etc., to help you both adjust calmly.
- Your birth experience is independent from having a healthy baby. It's important to seek support and get answers if your birth unfolded in an unexpected or difficult way.
- How you decide to feed your baby is a personal choice. Support is crucial for breastfeeding mums.
- Remember to rest, recover and process your journey into motherhood.

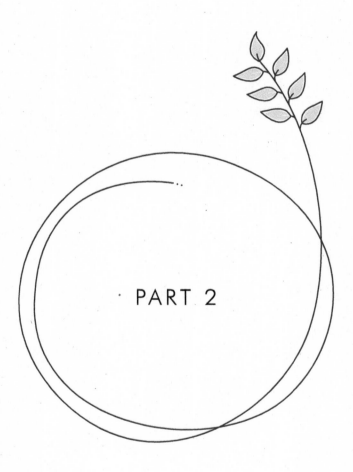

PART 2

Newborn to Three Months

The 'fourth trimester' is the nickname given to the first three months following birth. Postpartum/postnatal usually only refers to the first eight weeks after birth and is more of a medical term. Referring to these first three months as a trimester is possibly more relatable for mums, and viewing this time as an extension of pregnancy can set you up with a more realistic mindset. Of course, your baby is no longer inside your body, but **you are still very much sharing your body in many, many ways**; newborns are reliant on you and your body for everything, after all.

In this section we are going to run through some of the common challenges new parents face within those first three months, from the shock of becoming a parent to postnatal symptoms and newborn conditions. I've got some solutions and suggestions I really hope you find useful, but, as I'm sure you'd expect, I won't be able to cover absolutely everything here and you may experience several other changes or difficulties. Remember, there are professionals and experts who can help you. It's a case of identifying the problem or concern and finding the right person to help. As you'll go on to find out, I am a huge fan of delegating and it's how I get through a lot of my life when I'm overwhelmed. In general I delegate, automate or eliminate. When none of those is possible, I prioritise the problem or whatever it is that needs my attention specifically and try to get it sorted as soon as possible.

Your birth experience and baby's weight, temperament, genetics and any medical conditions will all impact your new family's experiences. For example, babies with a low birth weight may need feeding more regularly, which can be even more tiring for parents. Some babies' little personalities shine through early on – they will quickly let you know when they're not happy – whereas others are less bothered and more 'chilled' by nature. And finally, medical conditions or complications can impact early experiences for all; sometimes babies need to stay in hospital or be re-admitted for infections, jaundice, etc. Always seek individualised advice where necessary; you're never being a nuisance to anyone. I can promise you, the earlier you have discussions and raise any concerns, the better. These conversations will either reassure you things are normal or enable you to get specialised help. You deserve that at the very least.

We are going to start by exploring early experiences, and some mums will join us along the way and share their very honest accounts of motherhood.

Birth's the hard part . . . right?

SOMETIMES MUMS JOKE with me – they thought pregnancy and birth were the hard part, then they're faced with the fourth trimester. This time is often sprinkled with all kinds of new experiences, emotions, sensations, physical symptoms, relationship changes and shock. Some mums face challenges in those early months they may have never considered – with the birth having been at the forefront of their mind.

'I thought that I just had to get through the end of pregnancy and then birth and then it would get easier. This was so far from reality it's ridiculous. I had a very quick birth and left the birth centre seven hours later. I was on cloud nine – for about ten seconds. I very quickly realised I had no idea what I was doing. My daughter had a poo explosion, but I hadn't ever changed a newborn's nappy on my own. I carried her back into the hospital, trying to find the baby-changing facilities. She was screaming by this point and people were staring. It was embarrassing. I finally found the facilities and changed her. I got back to the car, but as soon as I put her in the car seat she started screaming again. We didn't know what to do. I almost went back into the maternity unit to ask the midwives. Fear of being judged stopped me. I was her mummy and I should know what to do. We got her in and out of that car seat about five times before we agreed to drive home regardless. She screamed the entire 22-minute journey. I tried singing and stroking her, but she got more upset so we sat listening to her scream in the end. We pulled up on the driveway and I broke down in tears as soon as I lifted her towards me. She was bright red and her tiny little body was shaking with stress too. I wondered if I had damaged her in some way. We've just got through the fourth trimester and things are getting easier and more predictable now. I really wish I had prepared more for motherhood and not just birth. I also wish I hadn't got so worked up and judged myself for everything from day one. That voice in my head was cruel at times. No one is perfect and parenting is learning on the job. As clichéd as it is, my advice is to be kind to yourself.'

Anonymous, first-time mum

It is very common for new parents to have an expectation of early parenthood that differs greatly from the reality of it. It's not your fault – we used to live in small villages or tribes, close to lots of women in our neighbourhood, but now we are perhaps more spread out, living in the digital age, and the experiences and wisdom of other mothers aren't passed down to us as they were before. Things you may never have had to think about suddenly become a big part of your life. The fact that babies are non-verbal and unable to really explain what they need for a couple of years or so means you need to either guess what they need or plan everything in advance – and it's *hard work*. Please don't think that makes you incapable or disorganised. Motherhood can seem chaotic. There is a lot to adjust to and, on top of that adjustment, you don't need any negative commentary, so try to keep on top of that inner voice early on. Instead, remind yourself of all the amazing things you have accomplished. Talk to yourself the way you would talk to a friend. Show yourself compassion and love in the moments of chaos. You're the best mum for your baby.

THE ROLLERCOASTER RIDE AND FINDING YOUR MUM TRIBE

Things move at a very fast pace and sometimes your baby's needs change from minute to minute. The demands of a newborn can feel like a bit of a rollercoaster for you, as they're very calm and quiet one minute and then suddenly upset the next. Many mums tell me they find this particularly hard – the unpredictable ups and downs, all the while not being able to communicate through language. It can be hard to focus on anything other than your baby because you know you may need to act quickly at any given moment. Lots of mums report feeling slightly 'on edge' during the fourth trimester (and sometimes thereafter) as they get to know their baby and help them understand this whole new world (as we saw in Part 1, pages 30–31).

If you are feeling slightly anxious or on edge, remember that your needs matter too and **it is important to calm your nervous system**. After birth, there is a lot of focus on the baby as you will have been discharged from the maternity team and had a six-to-eight-week GP check but then not a lot else. That is why you need to advocate for yourself, reporting anything that doesn't feel right, and not accepting 'That's normal, you've just had a baby' if you feel it's not. You also need to rest and implement the support you need. Rather than trying to get a few hours off to do something recreational, try to build in little daily things you can do – like ten minutes of stretching and breathing, or 20 minutes in the bath with music and aromatherapy oils. **It's the little things we do daily that make a difference overall**. The more you implement these moments of self-care, the more they become habitual. It took me quite a long time to get to this stage, but I now automatically factor in 'me time'. The difference this has made to my mental wellbeing is enormous as well as liberating.

Remember, you always have professional support available to you too, in the form of local groups or apps that are made for new mums, like Peanut, Mush and Mums Anywhere (see page 245). There are hundreds and thousands of other mums out there looking for support and, when you find a mum tribe, it can be such a relief to offload and have those honest chats – just like our ancestors used to many years ago.

'I just loved the fourth trimester; my baby was really chilled and didn't cry much unless he was hungry. Waking up in the night to feed him was tiring, but I can literally sleep anywhere at any time, so I'd sleep a lot in the day or just totally switch off and relax watching TV. The house got pretty messy at times, but I took the advice from your first book and asked the visitors to do their bit. They knew the drill after a few visits and I didn't have to ask anymore. He's 16 weeks now and it has got a bit harder as he's got older, actually. The visitors aren't as frequent or hands-on now, but he's still pretty chilled overall and we still nap together in the day, sometimes for a few hours. I never feel guilty for it!'

Jade, first-time mum

I think most of us could do with a little more of Jade's attitude in our lives. Anecdotally, her outlook and experiences are not the norm – yet they can be, especially when you get comfortable asking for help, delegating and surrendering to rest. We are encouraged to live at such a fast pace now, to reply to emails within minutes and to cram as much into our day as possible. Yet we have the right to rest, slow down when we feel the need to and take time out. If there's any time during your life when you need to rest, it's after undergoing the biggest physical and emotional transformation life has to offer: pregnancy and birth. Your organs have been displaced, your heart has pumped to the extent of an Olympic athlete (that's not an exaggeration – your blood volume increased and your body needs to readjust to get back to its non-pregnant state), not to mention the rather large internal wound every single mum has on her uterus – where the placenta has been housed. These vessels need to close over and your body needs to heal. If more mums were able to relax more, whether by getting the right support or allowing themselves to rest, I'm sure motherhood would be a slightly easier adjustment and leave mums feeling better able to process this transition. When I refer to rest, I don't mean sitting down all day, though, as gentle movement is part of a healthy recovery. But rest from society, social media, too many conversations and questions, a to-do list, etc., is a must.

INTRODUCING YOUR NEW BABY TO YOUR BIGGER BABY

If this is not your first baby, like many mums you may feel worried or even guilty when it comes to introducing siblings. How will they react? At the time of writing, I am about to go through this myself and the anticipation is real! Having met thousands of mums and witnessed first introductions on many occasions, I have seen a couple of approaches that appear to work really well.

Firstly, it's so important to explain to the older sibling that they are about to meet their baby brother or sister – of course making sure all information is age-appropriate – but you may also want to warn them in advance about Mummy, or how Mummy is feeling and what is happening with Mummy. They may not be able to express this, but they may notice any drips or anything 'abnormal' on Mummy and feel concerned or confused by this.

Another consideration is allowing your child to take the time they need to see the baby. Many kids don't like feeling a lack of control or being forced into an interaction. So explain and let them explore/meet the baby in their own time – there's no rush. Likely, the more you push them, the more they will resist.

Consider all the new products the baby may have and perhaps look to get the older sibling something too. My friend did this recently and it worked so well; her three-year-old was thrilled and thanked the baby!

Lastly, inclusion: this is an obvious one, but I've seen it done so beautifully on a few occasions. When siblings weren't too sure about the tiny newborn and were looking fairly unimpressed, Mum saying, 'Would you like to help me change the nappy?' or 'Could you pick an outfit for your baby sister? She needs some help!', then praising their involvement and letting them know what a lovely big brother or sister they are, shows them they are still a valuable member of the family who is trusted and capable of helping. If you constantly try to guard a newborn from an older child, it may make the sibling feel pushed out or less important than the new baby.

Ultimately, though, you know your child and how to work with them in this situation – what lights them up and what upsets them. So, as always, go with your gut and know that, if the first meeting doesn't go well, it means nothing at all about their long-term relationship.

'When Arthur met Charlie, well, he didn't meet him as he took no notice of him whatsoever! I was eating toast and he didn't even look at the baby – he just went for some of my toast! He then turned his attention to the birthing pool in the lounge and asked to have a swim. I did worry they wouldn't bond because he wasn't interested in him at all, but eight months in and they love each other. It's so lovely to watch their little interactions and making each other laugh.'

Holly, mum of two

The first 42 days

THE FIRST 42 days is a topic that comes up a lot when I speak to both expectant parents and new mums because this time after birth is globally recognised due to its importance. Before we delve into some really important ideas for you to consider on your journey, remember that all births in England, Wales and Northern Ireland must be registered within 42 days of the child being born.

In my first book (which focused on pregnancy, birth and beyond), I highlighted the various practices around the globe during the first 42 days following birth. Ayurvedic medicine ('Ayurveda' for short), often translated as the 'science of life', is one of the world's oldest whole-body healing systems and was developed more than 3,000 years ago in India. Although there's a lack of research into how effective some of the practices are, it remains a really interesting concept for me, as a clinician and mum. Many of the themes and focuses on caring for new mums in Ayurveda are found throughout the world. These focuses are often: rest, support, temperature (keeping new mums warm); nutrition that aids repairing and is healing, re-nourishing and easily digestible; and the use of herbs and massage to help the uterus to involute (shrink back to pre-pregnancy) and close the space that's been left within the body after birth. China, Mexico and India, to name just a few, all share similar concepts, but there are many cultures around the world that respect the postpartum period as a time of restoration.

'In our area of Morocco, the family is traditionally very involved in the upbringing of babies and it's a lot of women supporting women. People tend to live in very close family units so there are always people around. The extended family unit has a close bond that they don't always have in the UK.'

Shiraz, Amayour Surf & Yoga

It is believed by millions of people globally that the first 42 days after birth set you up for the next 42 years. So let's delve into that idea for a moment: **I truly**

believe your postpartum recovery is just as important as your health during pregnancy, and we just don't stress this enough in the Western world. We will go on to explore exactly why I think that from a biochemical and psychological perspective in just a moment. As you know, your health, identity and many aspects of your life are impacted after birth – on both a physical and an emotional level. It's important to know that during pregnancy and postpartum mental health problems can present for the first time. Issues you may have been able to suppress or rationalise can bubble to the surface. To further that, hormonal imbalances, sleep deprivation, managing any health complications, the stress of having to care for a tiny person, and nutritional deficiencies may also contribute to mental health problems. Sometimes these difficulties are short-lived and are resolved by solid, consistent emotional support, rest, focus on healing, attention to diet and consideration of supplements, movement or massage, and hormonal fluctuations stabilising. If you are able to really approach healing in those first 42 days holistically, it is possible mental health or emotional difficulties will be more manageable and perhaps shorter-lived or even barely noticeable. There is a lack of medical evidence to support this view because we tend to treat problems rather than prevent them – hence my careful use of the word 'possible'. We have far more research and even surveillance during pregnancy and birth, which may contribute to the focus we tend to have on those two events. Yet anecdotally I notice a very clear difference between mothers who have had the opportunity to really (whole-body) heal from birth and ease gently into motherhood and those who have not had this opportunity or the support they need to do so. Postpartum problems, such as incontinence, particularly peeing yourself, and general physical and emotional pain, have almost been normalised in our culture. I really want you to know that it's *not* normal to feel persistently bad most days – you deserve better.

Roughly 38 per cent of women diagnosed with PND found it becomes a life-long condition, according to a report published in the *Harvard Review of Psychiatry* in 2014. Another Australian study showed that the peak incidence of depression postnatally was shockingly around four to five years after the birth of a baby. This is possibly due to changing support as babies become children, as well as recurring mental health symptoms that become progressively worse over time.

Given all this, I really want to take this moment to remind you how important it is to set yourself up well, early doors, at this time in your life. Please give yourself permission to slow down and feel confident to ask for support – guilt-free. I know it's not easy to do this – I too struggled at times and ended up doing things I didn't really need to. Usually due to some nonsense I'd tell myself, like, 'You'd better get out of the house today because Georgie needs to be taken out for a walk,' when in reality she was four weeks old, so sitting in the garden or walking around, experiencing the sensation of wind, hearing the birds and seeing the bushes were all that was needed. I promise you, little tweaks to take the pressure off you to do things that aren't absolutely necessary make a huge difference during your recovery period. That said, on the days you feel up to it and ready for it, getting gentle movement back into the body is an important part of your recovery. Walking around, stretching, nice deep breathing and pelvic floor strengthening are so beneficial. Something else that may help is to try to say no to people or things you aren't up for.

Kat King, mentioned on page 27, was my yoga teacher and doula during pregnancy, but I also booked her for her postnatal services. I knew the value of having her support postpartum, as well as in the lead-up to and during birth. And my goodness was I glad I did book her for the postnatal period too! Not everyone has the budget for this and, to be honest, we were a little strapped for cash at the time (it was at the height of the COVID-19 pandemic and Andy couldn't work), so Kat and I came up with an arrangement that worked for both of us. Some doulas are happy to do exchanges for other services or goods – not just monetary. Kat did simple yet very helpful things, like filling up my fridge and freezer with food (more on postpartum nutrition in the next section).

Kat also performed a 'closing of the bones' ceremony (you'll learn more about this in a minute if you haven't heard of it before) and kept reminding me/ giving me permission to rest. I am my own worst enemy when it comes to rest – many of us mums are – but having Kat to keep enabling and encouraging me changed my self-chatter and did really help in those early weeks.

> 'After birth, a mother is left open – spiritually, energetically – and can be vulnerable. The whole process needs time. We are a society of "to do and consume". We need to change the norm of flowers and babygrows being the most common gifts. What mums really need are general household goods, meal vouchers, food deliveries, massages and sleep – for both parents. We underestimate how much rest is needed, and often feel guilty for "not doing". A tip I love is to wear PJs (you should buy some nice new ones) – this is a great visual to visitors that "I am still healing; I need sleep and rest." And if someone is outstaying their welcome or pushing an opinion, remember it's never too late to set boundaries.'
>
> Kat King, doula and yoga teacher, Loveuyoga

CLOSING OF THE BONES CEREMONY

This is a traditional practice originating in Mexico and includes the use of the *rebozo*, a hand-woven shawl that's often handed down from mentor to student midwife. The rebozo is also commonly used during birth to support optimal fetal positioning and relieve pressure on the mother's back and pelvis. Kat taught Andy how to use it and we have some great photos of him in action during the birth of Georgie. After birth, the shawl is used to wrap the mother's hips and massage her. This ritual is done around six times during the first 40 days after birth. The combination of massaging then wrapping the mother with specially chosen oils and herbs helps to stimulate blood flow, release fluids and hormones, and tone muscles.

The ceremony begins with the mother lying flat on a mat and the practitioner gently rocking her hips using the rebozo. This felt amazing when Kat did it for me – I felt so light and a sense of freedom. We had candles burning and music playing; I think that also helped to relax me further. Following that, the mother's belly is massaged with a comforting warm oil using an ancient technique.

The ceremony ends with 'closing the bones' and the mother's hips are tightly wrapped with the rebozo. As she lies wrapped, her hands, arms, face and feet are massaged. Each practitioner may do things in a different way: many then leave the room, some do reiki, drum or sing.

'This kind of body work is essential to pelvic floor care, putting the hips and pelvis back into the correct place. Once unwrapped, some mothers have a sense of being reborn themselves. But if this all sounds a bit "woo-woo" for you, perhaps have a think about regular postnatal body work and wearing a temporary support belt to aid the joints and ligaments.'

Kat King, doula and yoga teacher, Loveuyoga

It's a beautiful ceremony that recognises what a mother has been through to grow and birth a baby. It supports new mothers to have the opportunity to relax, restore and recover from birth.

There's more neurogenesis (the process by which new neurons are formed in the brain) occurring during pregnancy and postpartum than there is during adolescence. What this tells us is that your brain has changed a lot. The term for this, coined by anthropologists, is matrescence. In short, there is a lot going on in your brain as well as your body and because we can't physically see those changes, we can run the risk of ignoring them. In the Western world we have lost touch with what new mothers really need. Placing emphasis on fitting into your pre-pregnancy jeans again or getting back to 'normal' to be seen as a strong, independent woman who *can* and will do it all – all this is unattainable because, after birth, you never get back to 'normal'. Instead, you're an altered version of yourself, and that's a good thing and to be embraced. You get the opportunity to see the world in a different way and (hopefully) respect the power of your body to have grown a whole other conscious human. What you have done is a real-life miracle.

Here are a few suggestions to help support your recovery. Focus on:

- Those first 42 days after birth and creating a healing sanctuary for yourself.
- Rest, recovery and delegating all tasks someone else can do.
- Nourishing yourself by adding/including nutrient-dense foods/herbs and spices in your diet. (See pages 72–5 for more on this.)
- Reducing time spent with negative/self-centred people or anyone who doesn't energise you. Ditch the drainers: now is not the time for you to be an emotional crutch to anyone else.
- Reporting any concerns to the most appropriate specialist. Your GP may be able to signpost you if you're not sure.
- Getting gentle movement back into your body when you're ready. That can start with stretching, and be as simple as circling your ankles, standing and stretching your calves using the wall for support, and pelvic floor exercises.
- Going to bed early. I know how tempting it is to stay up late with your partner watching that extra Netflix episode, but it's just not worth it if you are up frequently in the night.
- Asking your GP about their care pathway to monitor your long-term health if you were diagnosed with a condition such as diabetes.

'"The first 40 days", "the lying-in period", "confinement" are all ways ancient traditions describe the practice and wisdom of nesting, resting and being close to baby for this transitional and frankly mind-bending stage in life! It's important to note here that, whatever stage of postpartum you are (ahem . . . postpartum is forever!), it's never too late to apply this practice to your daily life: slowing down and resting when your body signals exhaustion. Rest is a doing word.'

Kate Longden, chef, nourisher, kitchen coach
and founder of The Food Doula

Postpartum nutrition

DEPENDING ON YOUR set-up at home and your personal interests, you may or may not have thought about postpartum nutrition. Many mums look into all the foods to avoid and take every supplement recommended during pregnancy. Then they enter into the postpartum period and don't treat themselves or their bodies in the same way. Because they're no longer pregnant, they don't feel as though nutrition is as important as it was when they were carrying their baby. I think you can guess what I am about to say: this really isn't the case, and it's hard. Because you're an amazing mum and want to focus on your baby, you can forget yourself. But your nutrition and what you put into your body is as important as it was during pregnancy.

Your incredible body needs your help to recover; it needs fuel and nutrient-dense food, and to be loved and considered. You need to regain strength and replenish your body while it returns to its non-pregnant state. Many experts now recommend personalised nutrition and avoiding following ideas set by others, because how our bodies absorb and tolerate nutrients varies. You can start to implement this by simply noticing how you feel after eating certain foods – your body will often tell you what it likes and does not like. Intuitive eating helps you to build a longer-lasting, healthier relationship with your body than dieting ever will. We all lack motivation to choose the more nourishing option on some days and that's okay too; we don't need to punish ourselves about that. We just need to stay in tune with our bodies and keep noticing how we feel.

Traditional Chinese medicine and Ayurvedic postpartum wisdom recommend avoiding cold and raw food. Warm, slow-cooked, easily digestible foods, with warming spices, help to keep things moving and are gentle on the gut in early postpartum. Think soups, stews, curries, broths and herbal teas. This principle offers the digestive system a softer landing into slow and steady physical recovery.

STABILISING YOUR BLOOD SUGAR

I asked Kate Longden, founder of The Food Doula, about how to stabilise blood sugar and this is what she said:

'Pairing a complex carb with protein for any snack or meal protects blood sugars from spiking. Preventing spikes can help prevent sugar crashes. This principle, alongside including an abundant variety of plants and a good intake of healthy fats – extra-virgin olive oil, avocado, good-quality dairy, bone broth, oily fish, coconut oil, grass-fed ghee – will set you up to feel good and raise/maintain some energy.

'Complex carbs include: quinoa, oats, brown rice, beans, buckwheat, wholemeal pasta/bread, new potatoes. Proteins include: fish, meat, chicken, Greek yoghurt, pulses, edamame, eggs, tofu, chopped nuts, nut butter, seeds.'

Tip: Smoothies are a great source of easily digestible nutrients. Play around with combos and flavours such as: plant milk, some nuts, berries, any fruit, nut butter, oats, quinoa, coconut milk, spirulina powder, maca, cacao powder, honey, dates, cinnamon, nutmeg, turmeric, mint, basil, cucumber, spinach, kale, beetroot, seeds and Greek yoghurt.

NEW MUM FOOD HACKS

Below Kate shares some helpful tips to get maximum nutrition when you're short on time and energy:

- Roast some veg to have in wholegrain bread toasties – you cannot go wrong with a hot sandwich!
- Make some popcorn, then, when you're hungry, melt a bit of butter, add your favourite spices and mix into the popcorn.
- Stuff some dates with peanut butter and keep in the fridge or freezer for a quick snack.

- Chuck ingredients in the slow cooker in the morning, which will cook through the day, then you have your evening meal sorted, with almost no effort at all.
- Put ground or whole seeds and ground or chopped nuts in jars next to the salt and pepper so you automatically sprinkle some on each meal. Here are seven good options: flax, chia, linseed, pumpkin, sunflower, sesame and hemp.
- Avocado on toast is great, and even better with some protein. Add an egg, a sprinkling of the seeds listed above, lentils or some spiced yoghurt.
- Make a nutrient-dense smoothie the night before, so in the morning it is ready to go and provide you with a blast of goodness early on (see previous page for some good combos). Even better if someone can bring it to you in bed!
- Try to stack a food-prep habit on top of an existing kitchen habit, such as boiling the kettle or emptying the dishwasher – it can be a real game-changer. In the time it takes to make and drink your cuppa, boil some quinoa, rice, wholegrain pasta or new potatoes – these can keep in the fridge for a few days and accompany any meal.

WELLNESS EXPERTS AND MODERN MEDICINE

As you'll know, there are clinical doctors and holistic health practitioners, and I really value the expertise of both. Some mums prefer to speak to a doctor about any issues they face and prefer pharmaceutical treatment. Others prefer to seek holistic or alternative therapies.

It's good to bear in mind the severity of your situation and what *you* think you really need. Sometimes that will be a prescription, other times it may be a case of trying to pinpoint the root cause of any issues you're facing and seeking support for that before you opt for medical treatment. A combination of the two practices may also be really helpful and you don't need to 'pick a team'. They both have a place.

In my midwifery practice, I almost always opt for low-tech, minimal medication and intervention where possible, and aim to work with the body to reduce the problem, pain or emotion. Your body is incredible and sometimes a small tweak will offer it the support it needs to self-heal. Of course, there are occasions when I go straight for medication and I want to be really clear on the fact that we must not be dismissive of medical complications, but this is less common. If you do seek out any alternative therapies, ensure the person has decent experience and is registered with the appropriate authorising body – if there is one.

A NOTE ON VITAMINS

Currently, evidence regarding interventions that might prevent or treat PND is lacking. That said, I do believe a diet deficient in certain vitamins, minerals or other nutrients will likely impact symptoms in some women. Correcting this deficiency with dietary supplements might therefore prevent PND. Examples of possible dietary supplements aimed at preventing PND include: omega-3 fatty acids, iron, folate, s-adenosyl-L-methionine, vitamins B12, B6, B2, vitamin D and calcium.

Common symptoms

NOW WE ARE going to move on to the more practical stuff – the physical symptoms you may experience in the fourth trimester and things to avoid or try. Please don't be alarmed by the range of symptoms; some mums hardly get any of these and others get lots. Either way, we need to talk about them more.

CAN PREGNANCY HELP US UNDERSTAND LONG-TERM HEALTH?

This is a question I asked myself not long after qualifying as a midwife and is an area I became particularly interested in. Spoiler alert: my conclusion is yes, it is likely that pregnancy can help us improve long-term health by providing early warning signs. Here's why: pregnancy puts a tremendous amount of strain on the body. For evolutionary reasons, the body will protect a growing fetus at almost any cost to the mother, prioritising nutrition, among other things, to ensure the baby gets what the baby needs and has a decent filter (the placenta), all created and maintained by the mother's body. The physiological changes and symptoms you experience could therefore be early indicators of potential predispositions to certain health conditions. Some physical issues may resolve after birth never to be seen again or they can advance into chronic health problems later on. For example, mums who experience gestational diabetes or particularly high blood pressure/ pre-eclampsia are more likely to develop diabetes or cardiac-related health conditions later on in life. Due to the strain on the body, pregnancy and the postnatal period can cause underlying health issues to present for the first time. Knowing this may support mums by highlighting a need to focus on certain aspects to optimise health and happiness.

Understanding why these signs show up could be an opportunity to learn how to look after your unique self. You may be able to reduce the chances of conditions reappearing later on in life by making some simple lifestyle changes and understanding your body or environmental factors better, so I don't want you to feel scared by this. Having this knowledge can be a positive thing when you embrace the opportunity to listen to your body and take the steps you need to really heal from pregnancy and birth while optimising your future health.

NIGHT SWEATS

You may have already experienced night sweats during pregnancy – lots of mums get them in the first trimester. However, postpartum sweats are caused by changing hormones and rapidly decreasing amounts of oestrogen and progesterone. They can be worse for breastfeeding mums as these hormones stay low until you stop breastfeeding. Some mums have told me they wake up so wet with sweat they've have to get changed in the night. I didn't get sweats, but Andy couldn't cuddle me in bed because I 'pumped out heat like a radiator'.

Try:
- Using cotton pillowcases, light duvets or blankets. Temperatures have been rising in the UK and it's been particularly hot in the summer months. If it is too hot, try using a cotton sheet in place of your duvet and keep the duvet at the foot of the bed, ready to be pulled on if you want it.
- Wearing light, cool and breathable material like organic cotton that's loose-fitting, or getting as naked as possible, depending on your bleeding/milk-leaking situation.
- Keeping your vagina healthy. This is important, as allowing airflow down below can aid healing wounds and reduce your chances of developing thrush (see box over the page), just like nappy-free time helps reduce nappy rash soreness. Get some puppy pads, an old towel or something to put under you so you can have knicker-free time.
- Keeping a bottle of water next to your bed, ready to sip to help rehydrate you. Aim to drink around 3 litres of water a day, more if you had a heavy blood loss at birth.

Avoid:

- Using a static fan aimed directly at you and especially your baby (if you are co-sleeping/breastfeeding) as this can cause a drastic drop in temperature.

For most, night sweats will settle down after a few months, although they can persist longer for breastfeeding mums, as mentioned.

Note: Having a high temperature (pyrexial) or fever can be associated with infection. If you spike a temperature of more than 37.5°C or have any other signs of infection, such as feeling generally unwell, a fast heart rate, any red, sore or swollen areas (particularly around any wounds) and anything that smells 'offensive', as clinicians say, let your midwife/doctor know so they can properly assess you and treat if necessary. Infection can be anything from mild to dangerous. If you're unsure, always report suspicious symptoms.

A NOTE ON THRUSH

Most women will be familiar with the symptoms of thrush by the time they have a baby, but the most common ones are red, itchy/inflamed skin, pain during penetration and the wonderful cottage-cheese-like discharge. You may get one or all of these. Thrush won't self-resolve (like bacterial vaginosis may do – another very common vaginal infection), so it's important to get treatment for thrush as soon as possible, which is available in various forms, such as creams and pessaries, at almost all pharmacies.

CONTINUED BLEEDING AFTER BIRTH

This is a healthy, normal part of your postnatal recovery. The lining of your womb sheds, as it does during a period, as the placental site needs to heal and the blood vessels to close over. This can take a few weeks for some mums. I would recommend finding out how much blood you lost at birth by asking your midwife so you can support your personal healing. Blood loss of <500ml is deemed normal, yet for someone who is smaller than average or already anaemic that blood loss can be impactful and make you feel tired or breathless. It's therefore important to consider how your blood loss at birth may affect your recovery. Make sure you're getting enough iron in your diet (see below for some iron-rich foods) or consider supplementation if not (see page 81).

FOODS RICH IN IRON

- legumes
- dark leafy greens
- fish, especially salmon, sardines, tuna
- eggs
- red meat
- dark chocolate and dried apricots (a personal favourite!)

Any blood loss >500ml is considered abnormal or is classified as a postpartum haemorrhage (PPH). Your body may compensate very well after this blood loss and there's a lot of treatment available from your midwife/doctor. Once you're home it is very important that you monitor further blood loss, once again making sure you restore iron and fluid levels. Monitoring the amount, colour and smell of vaginal loss (or lochia, as midwives refer to it) is important for all new mums. As a rule of thumb, you shouldn't be soaking pads hourly. If you are, you need to speak to your midwife urgently. An unpleasant smell usually indicates infection – please never feel embarrassed to tell us about this, as infection can significantly delay your recovery. Early recognition and treatment are key. There's not much that midwives haven't seen or smelt before. The most important thing to a mid-wife is to ensure mums are well cared for and receive optimal treatment.

Bleeding will start to reduce and gradually change colour after the first week. If you are sitting for long periods (especially if breastfeeding), it's normal to feel a surge of blood loss or to pass smaller clots when getting up.

Try:
- Period pants. These can be a good option, especially at night (in addition to night-time pads if you want extra protection against leakages). I started using period pants and never looked back.

Avoid:
- Tampons, even if you've had a C-section. It's easy to forget about them with a new baby and you're less able to properly assess your bleeding.

Note: Sometimes, around day nine or ten after birth, mums experience a heavier bleed or the loss of large clots. This can be quite shocking, especially as it is hardly ever discussed, but this sudden and heavy loss is a fairly common issue. If you start to bleed heavily at home or lose big clots, you need to call the maternity emergency line. The bleeding can look a bit scary, but it's okay – there's a lot we can do to manage it.

POSTNATAL CONTRACTIONS: 'AFTER PAINS'

'After pains' are caused by contractions as your uterus involutes and shrinks back down. Women often describe the contractions as being anything from uncomfortable to very painful. After having Georgie, despite consulting lots of mums with after pains, I was shocked at just how strong they were. I reverted to my hypnobirthing breathing to help manage the discomfort.

Generally, the contractions are at their peak in the hours after birth and diminish gradually over the first few days.

After pains may start or become stronger when you breastfeed – this is due to nipple stimulation triggering the uterus to contract and is one of the reasons immediate breastfeeding can help with preventing a postpartum haemorrhage (see page 79).

Try:
- Taking painkillers to help ease after pains. Speak to your midwife or doctor first about what's best/safest for you.

EXHAUSTION

Although feeling exhausted is very common during the first year of your baby's life, it may not just be due to lack of sleep. It's really important to consider everything that may be making you feel more exhausted. Listed below are a few key medical reasons:

1. Recovering from pregnancy and birth – arguably the biggest physical task the human body goes through. You may have had

a long labour, not slept well towards the end of your pregnancy, or have a wound that is healing. This will make you feel tired and need to rest more.

2. Blood loss and anaemia – lots of us are great at taking our pregnancy supplements but forget to continue postnatally. Unless you have had a PPH, you may not have any blood tests after birth to check your iron levels. Yet you may have bled fairly heavily for some days, perhaps even a few weeks. Without blood tests, anaemia can go undiagnosed. Consider supplementing and requesting blood tests if you think you may be anaemic. I'm an ambassador for Active Iron and take their supplements myself because they're clinically proven and do not cause the usual side effects such as constipation and nausea. Another consideration is vitamin B12. If deficient, getting an injection can really help tackle fatigue.

3. Abnormal thyroid function – postpartum thyroiditis affects approximately 1 in 20 women within the first year following birth. It's most common in women who have type 1 diabetes or a family history/previous history of abnormal thyroid function. In postpartum thyroiditis, the immune system attacks the thyroid within around six months after birth. Symptoms may include tiredness, irritability, trouble sleeping and a fast heartbeat. Report any of these symptoms to your GP.

HAEMORRHOIDS (PILES)

You may have had the pleasure of these unpleasant protrusions during pregnancy, or they may have come on after a vaginal birth. Please try not to feel embarrassed or worried about them – they're common and it's estimated that around 40 per cent of women experience them.

Haemorrhoids, or piles, are swollen veins inside or outside the anus. The veins supplying blood to the area get congested just inside or get pushed outside the anus. Pressure from the uterus and the weight of the growing baby, as well as changes in circulation, contribute to their development, and constipation/straining can also encourage them, but often it's a combination of factors.

The veins appear like 'lumps' and can be visible. Internal haemorrhoids are not visible to the naked eye but can be really uncomfortable. Other symptoms of haemorrhoids are itching and mild bleeding.

Try:

- Eating a fibrous diet and drinking plenty of water to help prevent constipation. Prunes, prune juice, aloe vera and laxatives can help, though speak to a healthcare professional before taking laxatives in case there are any contraindications or other information you need to be aware of.
- Gently cleaning the area after you have gone to the loo. You may also have a sensation like you still need to poo – this is due to the pressure on the anus sending a message to say you still need to go, and it can get very irritating.
- Leaving a cooling wipe (such as one containing witch hazel or aloe vera) in your underwear for a few minutes after going to the toilet, to soothe the area.
- Using Anusol (haemorrhoid treatment) infused wipes, which are available over the counter.
- Having a warm bath. Consider adding Epsom salts depending on any wounds and healing progress.

Avoid:

- Straining, which can exacerbate them – hence why a high-fibre diet can help.
- Running, jumping and using weights until you are ready, though light exercise such as walking or yoga is recommended. Listen to your body and avoid overexertion.

The combination of haemorrhoids and wounds can be a challenge and make you feel a bit down or defeated. Remember, as time goes on, they can naturally shrink and sometimes disappear. If they do hang around, request a referral from your GP to a specialist to discuss your options. More often than not, as with anything, there are options.

THE SIX-WEEK POSTNATAL CHECK

Around six weeks after you've had your baby, you'll be offered a postnatal check with a GP. This is a top-to-toe assessment and isn't too dissimilar to the postnatal check midwives perform before discharging you. On some occasions, your six-week check is offered via a telephone call, which I do not believe is sufficient for what you need. Depending on how you feel, I'd advise having a face-to-face appointment and ensuring all your concerns are covered.

Feel free to request a blood test if you're worried about low iron levels (see box on page 80 on reasons for exhaustion). NHS Blood and Transplant report up to 41 per cent of postnatal mothers become anaemic. Get your levels checked if you think you need to.

You may also be offered a combined check for you and your baby. I'd recommend having two separate appointments so that you get the time you need to run through questions and have dedicated time just for you. Any wounds you would like assessing should be checked and you should leave feeling satisfied with the care you have received. As I have often stressed throughout this section, your postnatal health is incredibly important and must be addressed with the attention and seriousness it deserves.

RETURN OF THE . . . PERIOD

The timing around getting your period again varies. If you bottle-feed your baby (or use a combination of bottle and breast), it could be as early as five to six weeks after birth. If you are exclusively breastfeeding, it will depend on how often you feed – particularly at night. It's usually the night feeds that suppress ovulation. If you don't want to fall pregnant again, you still need to be careful if you've got a male partner and are sexually active (see overleaf). I have looked after many mums with surprise babies after being caught off guard thinking they aren't fertile. You may still be able to conceive before your period has returned because you ovulate before your bleed.

CONTRACEPTION

This can be a tough one for many mums, especially those who do not want to take hormone-based contraceptives. Personally, I do not get on with hormonal contraceptives either. Below is a list of all the options to consider:

- Barrier methods: male or female condoms – not everyone's cup of tea but liked by others.
- Lactational amenorrhoea method (LAM): where ovulation is suppressed due to the high levels of prolactin that are produced during exclusive breastfeeding. This is 98 per cent effective when:

  — your baby is under six months old
  — you're exclusively (or almost exclusively) breastfeeding day and night
  — your periods have not returned

(Note: I have looked after a lady who fell pregnant while all three applied when her baby was five months old.)

- Natural family planning/fertility awareness: this involves cycle tracking, cervical mucus and temperature monitoring, to name a few. You can use this method once your periods have returned. Fertility UK has a great website for you to refer to (see page 243).
- The mini pill: this is progesterone-only and advised for breastfeeding mums.
- Intrauterine methods: this is a coil and can be hormonal or copper. Speak to your midwife for more information on these.
- Contraceptive patch, implant or injection: it's best to discuss this with your midwife or GP first to see how suitable these are for you.
- The 'pull-out method': I have to be real and put this in here, although it's not technically a contraception method, as not many healthcare providers will discuss it. The pull-out method is where your partner literally withdraws his penis before ejaculating. This is not a reliable method, but it's often used. Around 5–20 per cent of women fall pregnant while using this method.

C-SECTION RECOVERY

~~~~

Recovering from a C-section may take longer than a physiological vaginal birth, though not in all cases. Having a C-section involves major abdominal surgery, which is sometimes overlooked because women have a baby to care for. Again, preventing infection is key to optimising recovery, alongside getting gentle movement back in the body. When I say gentle, I literally mean circling your ankles, stretching, pelvic floor exercises and deep breathing with focused intent. This helps you to lay strong foundations and rebuilds strength. You can start these from your hospital bed and continue for as long as you feel you need to before moving on to bigger muscle groups such as your glutes. If you have any concerns about your pain or need stronger analgesia please do not hesitate to speak to a doctor about this.

Tip: Speak to your midwife, doctor or a women's health physio about scar massage, a hugely beneficial therapy. It aids healing, as well as reducing discomfort and the build-up of tissue.

PAIN DURING SEX

~~~~

Although I didn't need stitches after having Georgie, I had some decent grazes and one in a very unfortunate place! I was worried about how sex would feel and whether it would still be as enjoyable. The grazes healed quickly and did not affect my sex life in any way, but I know this is not the case for all mums. Sometimes pain during sex does occur and can persist. This is not something you have to put up with or accept. Your sex life and pleasure matter.

The key for many couples is communication: telling your partner what you want and need. It's less common for women to say what they like in the bedroom, so this time can be a great opportunity to be more confident and vocal about what you like. (To the women reading this who did this pre-birth, go you!) Keep up that open and honest pillow talk. It's great for your sex life and why should you settle for anything other than what gets you going?

In terms of timeframes, this is very individual and dependent on the type of birth, the healing process and any delays with infection, and how you feel emotionally. Some people will give a timeframe of, say, six weeks. I prefer never to set these timelines. We are very used to having set times for things, deadlines or appointments and so on. We can subconsciously then feel pressure as those six weeks come to a close. The very last thing I ever want you to feel as a new mum is unnecessary added pressure. Just as I recommend later on in the book, regarding your baby's inner timeline and paying attention to that, I recommend the same for you – especially where sex is concerned.

If you're starting to feel like you might be ready, I'd suggest having a little feel first yourself rather than getting straight down to it. Use a water-based lubricant and place one or two fingers inside your vagina to see how that feels. Find what's comfortable and any areas that aren't. You may also want to try a little massage and have a feel of the tissue. If you do have a scar, there's a lot of research to support how massage helps reduce scar tenderness and aids healing. You do need to wait until the wound is completely closed over until you try this, though.

If you have any concerns, it is important to speak up and ask a trained, clinical professional to have a look. I know it may feel a little awkward asking someone to look at your vagina after birth, especially if you are still bleeding, but remember that clinicians do not look at vaginas like everyone else. For us, looking at a vulva/vagina or perineum is like looking at a hand. In fact, I know vaginas way better than hands and am far more comfortable talking about them.

Remember: pain during sex is not an issue you need to simply put up with and it's not just part of mum life. It is something that needs to be properly addressed. Sexual function is important for our relationships, self-esteem and sexual health.

HAIR LOSS

Hair loss after birth is normal and very common, yet this symptom can come as a real shock because mums aren't usually warned about it. My friend called me when her baby was a few months old and said, 'I'm seriously panicking – am I going bald?!' Even I had forgotten to warn her that this could happen, so I'm making sure I give you the heads-up. During pregnancy you may have noticed that your hair became thicker. This is common but it doesn't happen to all women. Hormone levels, in particular the thyroid hormone, progesterone and oestrogen significantly increase during pregnancy – some of them by up to nine times. This increase accelerates hair growth and affects its natural cycle. Basically, less hair falls out because your hair remains in the 'anagen' (growth) phase longer than normal, leaving you with more hair.

After you have your baby, the additional hair growth from pregnancy and the hair that didn't fall out starts to 'shed' once your hormone levels return to normal. Most of us lose around 100 hairs per day, but after giving birth you may find that you are losing as many as 300 hairs per day. This will eventually revert to the usual amount and **you will not go bald**, even if your hair appears to come out in clumps.

In medical terms, postpartum hair loss is mostly documented as 'postpartum alopecia' – if you want to look it up and do a bit more research into it. For most mums, shedding starts between two and five months after birth and continues for an average of two to six months.

Areas of hair loss vary, but are usually more pronounced in those associated with male baldness (exciting news that, I know). If you ever have the pleasure of seeing my hairline, you'll know exactly what I'm talking about – the classic M shape plus a bit of fluff along the line. Your hair will grow back and, although there's not one product or practice that is guaranteed to help, there are a few things you can do to support regrowth.

Try:
- Eating a healthy balanced diet including proteins, essential fatty acids and minerals (see page 75). Supplements you may want to consider starting or to continue taking are iron, zinc and copper, and vitamins A, C, D, E and B, including biotin.
- Being gentle with your hair. I used to be really rough with mine, pulling a harsh brush through it quickly in the morning, but mistreating your hair can impact the amount that falls out in one go. Try a softer brush and being a little gentler. It won't stop hair loss, but it may help you hang on to those hairs that weren't quite ready to shed.
- Hair treatments. Again, they won't stop hair loss, but they may improve the quality and health of your hair overall, and it's a bit of self-care. If you can, once a week, get a hair mask on and have a nice warm bath with some oils or bath salts once any wounds have healed. You deserve it.
- Calming your nervous system, downregulating and resting. Deep breathing and gentle movement, such as walking or yoga, can help. We can't be certain this is related to humans, but high cortisol levels in

sheep are associated with increased postpartum hair loss. We also know stress is associated with hair loss in general. Yet another reason to ask for help and rest whenever you have the opportunity.

As I touched on earlier, sometimes symptoms presenting during pregnancy and the postnatal period can indicate other areas you need to pay more attention to. For prolonged and excessive hair loss those areas are:

- nutrition, and deficiencies
- very low-calorie intake/undereating
- stress
- thyroid problems

SWOLLEN LABIA

Many women (and men) do not have a complete understanding of female anatomy and female reproductive health. Shockingly, the clitoris was only discovered in its entirety in 1998 (yes, 1998 – can you believe that?) and some medical diagrams still display it incorrectly. Female reproductive health is something, as parents, we need to talk to our children and teenagers about – both male and female.

Labia – from the Latin word *labium* for lip – are the folds of skin around the entrance to your vagina. Labia majora are the outer lips and labia minora are the inner lips (which are inside the labia majora). The size and appearance of the labia minora vary from woman to woman, some bigger, some smaller, some sitting within the labia majora, some outside.

Mild to moderate postpartum swelling is very common, with some mums noticing labial swelling during pregnancy. This is usually nothing to worry about and it's caused by the pressure/weight of your baby and/or any trauma to your perineum while pushing your baby out. It tends to last a few days and then gradually subsides. If the swelling is becoming worse or not subsiding after one week, it could indicate infection or a haematoma (a collection of clotted blood) and both need to be addressed urgently and reported to your midwife or doctor.

On that note, if you have *any* concerns, *any* time, regarding your perineum, vulva, labia, vagina, anus, etc., please let your midwife know as soon as possible and do ask them to have a look.

Try:

- Cold packs wrapped in a towel or pillow case to help reduce the swelling. Some companies now sell pads that have inbuilt cooling gels that become cold once activated.
- Lavender baths. These are clinically proven to reduce pain and swelling.
- Resting on your side as and when you can. This will help you to heal and take the pressure off your pelvic region.
- Analgesia.

Avoid:

- Standing or sitting in one position for long periods.
- Douching. This is not good for healing and it can interfere with the very finely tuned bacterial ratio, causing imbalances such as bacterial vaginosis.
- Blow-drying your vulva after a shower or bath. There's a lot of advice floating around online about why this is good – it's not and it can cause any stitches you may have to break down quicker. It's best to dry yourself with a clean towel or let air get to your perineum (see page 77).

POSTPARTUM HEAVINESS IN THE PELVIC REGION

It's common to feel a sense of aching, dragging or heaviness from the vagina and pelvic region in general after birth. Feelings of heaviness are usually due to trauma/swelling/pushing and simple gravity. If you had a long vaginal labour and birth and/or had intervention, such as a ventouse (vacuum) or forceps, it's more likely you will experience this within the early weeks after birth.

If you notice any signs of prolapse – seeing a lump or bulge coming from your vagina (anything hanging down where it shouldn't be) – speak to your midwife or doctor as soon as possible.

Try:

- Resting when you can.
- Pelvic floor exercises as soon as you feel able to. I promise you, pelvic floor exercises make a huge difference. Doing them regularly will improve sexual function/pleasure, reduce discomfort and aid recovery.

Avoid:
- Standing for long periods – this can really make it worse until you've healed and regained strength in the pelvic floor.

OTHER POSTNATAL EXPERIENCES

Now that we've covered some of the physical changes after birth, we'll run through some of the neurological changes, including the reason you may find yourself jumping out of the shower, running to your baby soaking wet, only to find they are sound asleep.

Increased noise sensitivity

A postpartum symptom, due to neurological changes, is increased hearing or noise sensitivity. This is very rarely spoken about and I had never come across it before having Georgie. In my first book, I wrote about brain changes and the increased ability women have to read body language (due to changes in the grey matter of the brain), but I did not know about hearing changes post-natally at that time. These changes after birth are due to the fact that we are hardwired to nurture, care for and respond to our baby's needs . . . which is lovely, but an unexpected symptom and something that caught me off guard.

HONESTY BOX

I have always been sensitive to the noise generated by Andy's open-mouth eating – instant rage – but I noticed a big change in noise sensitivity after having Georgie. Noises I could usually tolerate and combinations of noises became difficult. For example, if the radio was on, Andy was talking and my phone started ringing, I'd feel overwhelmed and become unable to talk or focus. The sound of Georgie crying was by far the worst – it was so loud to me that I would describe it as almost painful at times. Her cry still goes through me and induces a stress response as soon as it's detected by my pinna (the portion of the outer ear collecting sound waves). This extreme reaction has calmed down throughout the first year of her life. The difference between Andy's and my response to her crying was remarkable. He could block it out and finish a conversation. However, I *had* to immediately respond and couldn't hold further conversation or process any information until I had done so. In fact, if someone dared to try to continue a conversation while she was crying, I'd become irritated. Yet the sound of babies crying is something I am well used to, both as a big sister and a midwife of many years. I would hear babies crying almost every time I walked into work, on and off throughout the 12–13-hour shifts, day and night. Therefore, I developed the ability to switch off from it when required. But not with my own baby – this was a totally different ball game.

Unsurprisingly, there hasn't been a huge amount of research into this increased noise sensitivity. It's the same old story – research into women's health has not been, and still isn't, given the attention it deserves, but let's not get into that now! Focusing on the positive, the research we do have is interesting and confirms my initial suspicion. My hearing had significantly changed after birth due to brain changes, and it is a symptom lots of new mums experience. One study found that, after birth, tissue increases within auditory areas. It's also thought these observed effects are related to the mother's brain changes, helping her to interpret her newborn baby's cries – almost like an inbuilt new-born translator. Pretty amazing, isn't it, the extent the body goes to in order to help us protect our babies?

Something else to bear in mind is how sleep deprivation impacts hearing. Another study found that high levels of emotional exhaustion increase sound sensitivity. In this study some people found fairly low volumes of sound, such as a conversation, uncomfortably loud. An important consideration here, as a result of this study, is how noise sensitivity may relate to postnatal depletion or depression. If you are struggling with hearing changes, please do speak to your midwife. It may be an early sign that you are depleted and they may be able to offer some solutions to support you.

Phantom crying, especially in the shower
I recently did a question box on Instagram and asked mums: 'What is or was the most shocking symptom you experienced after birth – that no one warned you about?' The responses were mostly night sweats, heavy bleeding, after pains, breastfeeding and – you guessed it – phantom cries.

Yet again, this very common experience is rarely discussed. So why do so many of us hear phantom cries? Especially in the shower! There are a few reasons: after birth you are responsible for a vulnerable human. You take this new role very seriously and do what you can to protect your baby. Although to you it may feel like your body and brain are doing the exact opposite, these symptoms are intended to support, protect and nurture you both. As a new mum you need to promptly respond to your baby's needs because they are so vulnerable. Your body does what it can to increase your ability and need to act. It is also very common for people who are in other situations where they need to acutely respond to some kind of stimulus to experience phantom noises. For example, a lot of my colleagues, myself included, hear patient buzzers or bleeps going off even when we aren't at work or on call. I would sometimes hear a buzzer just as I was falling asleep after a stressful night shift. My brain was still alert and stimulated, picking up on any noise that would mean I needed to act quickly and potentially save someone's life.

When you're in the shower your senses are altered, so you're hyperaware of what could be happening while your hearing is compromised. This is not a conscious thought; instead, it is a protective mechanism as your brain goes through changes to ensure you're able to cut through noise and pick up on your baby's cues.

The good news is, this is not something you will experience forever and it usually subsides as your baby becomes more independent and you relax into your role and routine. I do still hear phantom cries while Georgie is in nursery. In fact, I heard one while writing the previous chapter. They can be frustrating and suddenly impact your nervous system, alerting you for nothing, but they do become less frequent and less alarming as time goes on.

All new parents experience some level of anxiety, it's totally normal. Yet frequent or particularly loud phantom cries can be a sign of postnatal anxiety and can provoke or worsen existing anxiety. If you are having difficulty showering or doing anything that requires you to be apart from your baby for a short period of time without hearing phantom cries, it's probably worth having a chat with your GP, health visitor or midwife. Maternal mental health is vitally important to look after, and the sooner you seek support, the sooner you will start to understand yourself and how to manage symptoms and feel more confident.

Mental health in the fourth trimester

MENTAL HEALTH AND mental illnesses are huge topics individually, and it's only fairly recently that some of the taboo surrounding them has lifted and we've discussed mental health diagnoses more openly. Here we will explore some of the things you can do to support good mental health, but also understand how to identify when you may need to seek support.

Mental health is something we all experience and it is on a spectrum. We are usually able to identify when we feel well, when we feel like ourselves and are able to manage the ups and downs of life, and when we don't. It's normal to have bigger highs and lower lows in motherhood, though, especially within the first year. **There is so much to adjust to**: hormones, physical body changes, brain changes, sleep deprivation, relationship changes, career concerns (not for all but for many) and, as we know, sadly trauma for some mums. Due to the range of problems mums face and the many variables involved with mental health, I won't be able to cover everything in great detail here. What I will do is run through the most common questions I am asked and hopefully this will support you to identify issues for yourself.

THE HISTORY OF POSTPARTUM CARE

Before we get on to those, though, I just want to mention the history of how new mothers were treated around the seventeenth century and the 'blackout' period – a time when new mothers remained in darker rooms to recover and heal from birth. The length of their stay in a darkened room would depend on their birth and overall health. If a mum lost more blood, the blackout period would be longer than for a mum who had fewer complications and felt ready to return to the light of day again.

Mothers had a group of women around them, consisting of the midwife and the 'gossips', who had been specially invited to their birth and to their home after birth to support them. Men left the area and were not allowed to enter the room where a mother was giving birth or recovering from birth. The supporting group of women would black out the windows upon their arrival ahead of the birth, and would help new mums with things like laundry, caring for other children and cooking after the birth.

The point I want to highlight here is how much postpartum care has changed for us mums today: how mums are praised in the media for 'bouncing back' with a 'washboard stomach weeks after birth'; or are perhaps, in some instances, perceived as strong, independent and somehow more able if they take minimal rest and get back to 'normal' as quickly as possible. I did mention at the start of this section how the first 42 days impact mothers and how I have seen first-hand the huge benefits of whole-body healing at a slower pace when mums have been supported to do this (see pages 66–71). I do not believe that mental illnesses are solely down to environment and lack of support or pressure to rush recovery. However, I do think that environment, support and physical recovery always impact mental health in some way. All new mums need support, love and relief from daily life – not unrealistic expectations. I think we can learn a thing or two from history and the care women received all those years ago.

THE DIFFERENCE BETWEEN BABY BLUES AND POSTNATAL DEPRESSION (PND)

The main difference between baby blues and PND is usually the length of time you experience symptoms. Baby blues is a term often used to describe how new mums feel very early on in motherhood, usually presenting around days three to five, when there's a significant change in hormones – especially for breastfeeding mums. Mums often feel tearful, sometimes low, and have mood swings from pure love and joy to suddenly feeling overwhelmed or nervous. These typically last for less than two weeks and tend to be a very normal response to becoming a mother in this day and age.

Try to explore what it is you are feeling and sit with the emotion while it's there; talk to someone who loves you about it or let it all out and have a good cry. If you are able to do this it's more likely you will feel a little more in tune with yourself and have more self-compassion. When we start to judge ourselves and add on stories like 'I must be weak, everyone else looks like they've got it together – why am I crying all the time?', we tend to create a disconnect and spiral into negative thinking traps. If you start doing this, simply try to be aware of it. Observe your thoughts and unfair tag-along stories. Then try, where possible, to change any negative self-talk into a more positive narrative. Talk to your self like you would talk to a friend. And remember, what you have been through is tough – you're doing amazing!

PND is different and requires a different approach. Feeling low, experiencing a loss of interest in things that usually make you happy, having feelings of deep sadness and disconnect, withdrawing from social interactions and having difficulty bonding with your baby are all common symptoms. These tend to last for more than two weeks, unlike baby blues, and can start anytime during the first year. Many people think that because they don't get these symptoms in the first few months but they do later on, they can't have PND. In fact, this can and does happen later on, which is why it's important to identify it and seek help as soon as you're able to. Your GP and health visitor can help, as well as many charities (see page 244). Mama, I can sincerely promise you one thing about PND – it is **not** your fault. Your baby will not be taken away from you. You need the right support and you'll feel well again. This is not the new you and it is not just something you need to accept.

In general the options for you are:

- Psychotherapy and cognitive behavioural therapy (CBT): these are brilliant options to start with if your depression is identified earlier. Having the time out to talk and unpack your thoughts in a safe space with someone who's specifically trained to help you can be tremendously beneficial as well as relieve symptoms. I have seen many mums enter into therapy in difficult places and seen a new person come out of therapy. Even if you don't have depression, talking therapy can be a great way of getting to know yourself and dealing with any issues you may have, from childhood, trauma or past experiences.
- Medication: not everyone wants to take medication, and I do believe that it's best to try other methods where possible, such as self-help or psychotherapy. That said, if PND is progressed or severe, medication may be the first, safest and best option. Then reducing dosages and

looking at other options may be a good idea once mums are feeling better and more in control of their thoughts and feelings. PND can make mums feel out of control and as though they don't know who they are anymore. If you experience this, I promise you are absolutely capable of feeling more in control and well again. Seeking support is the first step to your recovery. Know that any medication prescribed will be safe to take if you're breastfeeding, but feel free to double-check before taking anything.

INTRUSIVE THOUGHTS

These are very common throughout the first year of your baby's life and beyond. They are disturbing thoughts that pop into your head and can be as straightforward as 'If I fall down the stairs I might fall on top of my baby' to upsetting thoughts about abusing or even sexually assaulting your baby. Yes, horrifying I know, but they happen to many amazing mums who love their babies dearly and would never, ever do such a thing. Which is why I want to be very open and honest with you about these thoughts: they do **not** define you, mama. The fact that you feel horrified demonstrates that these are intrusive thoughts and not desires. And, to reiterate, an intrusive thought feels out of character because they are not reflective of what you plan to do or are capable of doing. These thoughts are, believe it or not, a defence mechanism aiming to protect, similar to anxiety. Intrusive thoughts can be associated with postnatal anxiety, which we will get on to in just a moment.

One of the best ways to handle intrusive thoughts is by talking about them to someone you trust and acknowledging them. The more horrified you are and the more you try to push them away, mums report, the more they seem to appear and escalate. This takes practice but try to acknowledge the thought and avoid being driven by the emotion it evokes. Your internal dialogue may sound something like: 'That's a horrible intrusive thought I just had. It's not going to happen. I'm just trying to protect my baby from all eventualities: my baby is safe.' If you're finding these thoughts difficult to manage and they're impacting your life, please do speak to your doctor or midwife. Psychotherapist and author Anna Mathur is also is a great source of information and support, and shares a lot of free advice online, some of which has really supported me (see page 244).

HONESTY BOX

Andy and I suffered with horrible intrusive thoughts; some way worse than others. Andy started to shake his head when he got them and I knew he was having intrusive thoughts if I saw him do this. It was a way of trying to shake the thought out of his head and bring him back to reality. For us, violence or disturbing videos sometimes circulating online made these thoughts worse. We used to love a murder documentary, but this made our intrusive thoughts worse so we now focus on watching comedy instead. Over time, they have improved but they do still, to this day, randomly appear and can be upsetting. I now take a moment to think about what the thought is trying to tell me and ask if it has a purpose. Sometimes it's yes and maybe I do something different to make me feel safer; sometimes it's no and I move on – acknowledging it but not dwelling on it.

ANXIETY

Alongside PND, anxiety is the most common mental health problem new and expectant mums face. This is also reflected in the general population, with anxiety reaching record-level highs. Triggers and severity vary significantly and I have my own theories on why anxiety is increasing so much, mostly in relation to societal expectations, status and technology/social media. In new motherhood a certain amount of anxiety is to be expected – you're entering into the unknown. Even if you're an expert, all babies are different and come with their own personalities, needs, etc. I have cared for paediatricians who have reported that all their knowledge meant nothing when they had their own baby and they too found the feeling of lack of control difficult. You're not alone if you feel like this. We can't predict what will happen in the postnatal phase and our entire lives suddenly feel as though they're run by this tiny human: when you get to sleep, where you go, when you shower, and so on. Anxiety can manifest itself in unexpected ways: you may not want people to hold or touch your baby and you may feel very protective of them, becoming distressed if someone crosses your boundary. I had a home birth and had to take Georgie to be admitted into hospital to have treatment for jaundice. This was massively anxiety-provoking, as we had gone from our safe bubble at home, where I was more in control, to having to have her under light therapy, being unable to hold her when I wanted, and people coming in and out of my room, handling her and taking blood tests. Even as a clinician myself who's worked for years on wards and is comfortable in a clinical environment, I still found it invasive and I even brought her to the toilet with me as I didn't want to leave her or for anyone to pick her up/touch her without me there.

As I said above, triggers do vary, but a common theme with anxiety is feeling out of control. When we do not know what is going to happen next, sometimes our mind fills in the gaps with 'what ifs'. This is our brain's attempt to prevent harmful things happening to us or our babies. It does serve a purpose and can be helpful in protecting us, but the balance can tip and the anxiety itself may then become more harmful than any potential threat, leading to physical symptoms. These are usually a fast heart and breathing rate, repetitive thoughts, sweating, repetitive checking, difficulty focusing or being present in the moment, and changes in appetite. Anxiety may lead to a panic attack and can be very scary for the person experiencing it as they are literally living out their fears. Having seen some mums go through this, it's heartbreaking to watch a thought begin in the mind and reach significant physically visible levels of distress. Anxiety can be gripping and require professional support.

There are some incredible self-help options to start with if symptoms are milder, and pharmaceutical help in the form of medication too. If you notice a change in your thoughts and behaviours, or any of the physical symptoms described, know there's ever so much support available to you. All you need to do is reach out, to your GP or the charities featured in the resources section (see page 244).

POSTPARTUM RAGE

~~~~~

Although this is not recognised in its own right as a mental health condition, it's a common issue mums face and are rarely informed about. This may be due to the fact that it's not screened for or measured, but it's real. Postnatal rage is a thing and you're not alone if you get it – I experienced it too.

You may find you have angry outbursts, leading to you verbally lashing out at someone, irritability, or more physical manifestations such as breaking or throwing things. Some experts believe postpartum rage is due to feelings of powerlessness, while others believe sleep deprivation is to blame and some say it's probably hormonal. I think it's likely a combination of all. Although anger may also be associated with other mental health problems such as depression and anxiety, I don't believe postnatal rage is only ever a symptom of these conditions. I think you can have postnatal rage and not be depressed or anxious. If you get it, where possible try to identify triggers and manage them or stay away from them for the time being. If you think feelings of powerlessness are to blame, create a little (very little) to-do list and cross the things off that you've achieved that day. Seeing it written down can help you feel as though you have some control over the day and achieved the things you needed to – this really helped me when I felt overwhelmed and irritable. Cancel visitors if you need to rest or ask them to help so you can take a nap or do something for yourself, even if that's simply a shower or bath (see page 16 for a list of ways visitors can help). Always remind yourself at the end of the day that caring for a tiny human is one of the hardest yet most important jobs in the world. You're doing so, so well.

Night rage is similar – sudden intense anger – and may come as a shock. This type of rage usually occurs as a result of your state of being when asleep, which is driven by your parasympathetic nervous system. During sleep you're in the 'rest and digest' phase. When woken, suddenly the activation of the sympathetic autonomic nervous system is triggered. This system is basically your 'fight or flight' response – it's your body's natural defence mechanism and enables you to think fast and deal with an intruder, for example. So you go from being in a state of calm relaxation to being flooded with a sudden rush of stress hormones. In that moment it's therefore possible you'll feel some sort of rage, frustration or desire to run away. I've been there plenty of times, mama; it's not just you being unreasonable if you too experience this very valid emotion after being woken up. Where you are in your sleep cycle may affect how strong you experience these emotions.

To help calm your body down again, take a deep breath before you get up. Remind yourself of what has just happened and be kind to yourself. Ask for help – if you have someone you can share the night's wakings with, please do. When Georgie was around 12 weeks old, a little sleep hack I found helpful was going to bed at 8pm and getting Andy to give her a bottle of expressed milk at 10pm and then bring her up to bed. Sometimes she would wake at midnight, sometimes it was 2am. Either way, it meant I could get between four and six hours of solid sleep. I still felt rage when I was woken, but getting those solid hours in was helpful and did enable me to go into a deep sleep knowing I wouldn't be woken for some time.

Safer sleep for babies

I VOLUNTEER AS an ambassador for The Lullaby Trust, which has been running for over 50 years (see page 245). It's a wonderful charity that raises awareness of sudden infant death syndrome (SIDS, or cot death), provides expert advice on safer sleep for babies, and offers emotional support for bereaved families. I am so very grateful charities like this exist and I am happy to support the sharing of their messages to improve sleep safety. Their team have kindly contributed the words on the next few pages specially for this book. I hope you find the following helpful:

Safer sleep advice from The Lullaby Trust
The information here about safer sleep has saved many babies' lives. It is all backed by research that has shown how to reduce the chance of babies dying suddenly with no explanation. To reduce the chance of SIDS, families should follow this key advice for baby sleep. It is important that all parents and anyone involved in the care of a baby are aware of this advice:

- Put them on their BACK for every sleep.
- In a CLEAR, FLAT, SEPARATE SLEEP SPACE.
- Keep them SMOKE-FREE day and night.

Always place your baby on their back for sleep
- Put your baby down on their back – not their front or side – for every sleep.
- No special equipment or products are needed to keep them on their back.
- Once they start to roll from front to back by themselves, you can leave them to find their own position for sleep.
- Tummy time while awake can help to strengthen the muscles they need for rolling (see page 110).

Give your baby a clear, flat, separate, safe sleep space, in the same room as you

The safest place for a baby to sleep is in their own clear, flat, separate sleep space, such as a cot or Moses basket.

Whatever space you choose, follow these guidelines:

- A firm, flat mattress with no raised or cushioned areas.
- No pillows, quilts, duvets, bumpers or weighted bedding.
- No pods, nests or sleep positioners.
- Make sure your baby's head is kept uncovered so they don't get too hot. Try to keep the room temperature between 16°C and 20°C so that your baby does not get too hot or cold, and make sure bedding is appropriate for the time of year.
- Place baby at the bottom of the cot so that they cannot wriggle under covers – this is called 'feet to foot'.
- Ensure that the sleep space is kept clear of all items and there is nothing within reach of the space, for example, blind cords, nappy sacks or soft toys.
- Babies should always be in the same room as you for the first six months for sleep, day and night. This doesn't mean you can't leave the room to make a cup of tea or go to the toilet, but for most of the time when they are sleeping they are safest if you are close by.
- Babies should not be allowed to sleep in bouncy chairs and babies should not be left sleeping in their car seat when not travelling in the car. Car seats are not to be used as sleep spaces in the home.

Remember: if using a sleeping bag, no extra bedding is needed.

We are aware that not all parents are able to sleep their baby in a separate sleep space; for example, circumstances like fleeing from conflict or crisis mean that sleeping conditions will be unpredictable. It may not always be possible to access a recommended sleeping space for a baby, so we have adapted safer sleep advice based on different sleeping situations. Please refer to The Lullaby Trust advice and resources on their website for more information (see page 245).

Keep your baby smoke-free before and after birth

- Smoking in pregnancy greatly increases the chance of SIDS – all pregnant women should make every effort to take up the help to stop smoking provided locally.

- You should also avoid being exposed to others' smoke when you are pregnant – if your partner smokes, they can get help to quit too.
- Keep your baby away from smoke in your home, car and out and about.

Breastfeeding
- Breast milk and breastfeeding provide all the nutrition your baby needs for the first six months and protects them against infections and diseases.
- Breastfeeding lowers the chance of SIDS.

If you need more help with breastfeeding, talk to your midwife or health visitor or call the National Breastfeeding Helpline (see page 242). [If you are unable or do not want to breastfeed, see pages 47–51.]

Bedsharing more safely
Whether you choose to bedshare or it is unplanned, there are some key things you should avoid. It is dangerous to share a bed with your baby if:

- you or anyone in the bed has recently drunk any alcohol
- you or anyone in the bed smokes
- you or anyone in the bed has taken any drugs that make you feel sleepy
- your baby was born prematurely (before 37 weeks of pregnancy) or weighed under 2.5kg (5.5lb) when they were born

In these scenarios, it is always best to put baby in their own safe sleep space, such as a cot or Moses basket. Keeping the cot or Moses basket next to the bed might make it easier to do this.

Things to remember if bedsharing
- Keep pets away from the bed and do not have other children sharing the bed.
- Try to make sure or check that baby cannot fall out of bed or get trapped between the mattress and the wall.
- Keep pillows and adult bedding away from baby.

You should also follow the tips above if you think you might unexpectedly fall asleep with your baby in the bed (for example, during a night feed).

Never sleep with your baby on a sofa or armchair
- Sofas and armchairs are dangerous places to fall asleep with your baby – move somewhere safer if you might fall asleep.

Think ahead

Babies need a sober carer to be able to respond to their needs. Sometimes alcohol and drugs like cannabis and even some medicines make this harder for carers to do so. Planning ahead to have another adult like a partner or a close family member around to take care of the baby can be a good idea for those times. It's also really important to plan for babies to sleep in their own safe separate sleep space, such as a cot or Moses basket, if their carer has had any alcohol or drugs, or if they smoke.

Remember: if you think your baby is showing any signs of being unwell, always seek medical advice. The Lullaby Trust Baby Check app can help parents or carers determine how ill their baby is (see page 245).

MAKING THE DECISION TO CO-SLEEP

Thinking about Georgie's sleep needs really made me think about my own sleep needs. I co-slept with my parents until around the age of four, when I was finally happy to go in my own bed. Their bed was always available if I wanted to get in – usually after a nightmare or if I just needed a cuddle. I remember it well and the feeling of safety as I climbed in. Now, as an adult, I like going to bed at the same time as Andy and if he wants to stay up later it takes me longer to fall asleep alone. If I wake up in the night on my own, I feel uneasy. I am certainly more alert when alone at night. I do wonder if my sleep habits as a child have influenced my adult preferences. That said, I know many people experience the direct opposite. Lots of people like their own space and find that overheating or quilt-stealing inhibit a good night's sleep. Scientists have looked at the quality of sleep in couples who co-sleep. One study published by the American Academy of Sleep Medicine concluded: 'Sleeping with a partner was associated with lower depression, anxiety, and stress scores, and greater social support and satisfaction with life and relationships. Sleeping alone was associated with higher depression scores, and lower social support and life and relationship satisfaction.'

Interestingly the same study also brought attention to the impact of sleeping with children, stating that this was associated with more stress – a point that we will move on to in a little while, and I can absolutely vouch for! I co-slept with Georgie on and off for two years. As you'll read later in the book, we had a very tough time with sleep – Georgie woke very frequently and it wasn't always for food. But I'm not sure how else we could have managed to get any sleep or breastfeed for so long if we hadn't co-slept. Getting out of bed to go to her, or sitting up and manoeuvring around to get her closer or on the breast, repeatedly throughout the night, wasn't an option for me. Yet her restlessness in the night did disturb me often – or a fist to the face (always a nice wake-up call, that one!). Co-sleeping really was a double-edged sword and I had a love–hate relationship with it.

Henning Johannes Drews, a researcher at the Center for Integrative Psychiatry and a professor at the Department of Psychiatry and Psychotherapy at Christian-Albrechts University, Kiel, Germany, studied 12 heterosexual couples who spent four nights in a sleep lab – not a large sample size, but still really interesting to study. He concluded that sleeping together enhances REM sleep, which then may go on to reduce emotional stress and improve our interactions. He did also note this is subjective, stating, 'If your partner hinders you to fall asleep or disturbs your sleep, and you are much more relaxed if you sleep alone, that is probably the best sleeping arrangement to do.'

There is so much conflicting advice alongside some very strong opinions, with some saying that co-sleeping may impact healthy adult sleep habits and others that co-sleeping builds healthy strong bonds for life. Overall, sleep is subjective and easily impacted in the case of both adults and babies. Some of us have higher sleep needs than others. No one has an answer or method that works for everyone. If you choose to co-sleep, ensure you follow the safer sleep guidelines above.

'Frequent wake-ups are very normal for infants and it's important you respond to your baby's needs. If you are finding this difficult to manage, we would suggest talking to your health visitor about co-sleeping safely. For many parents this can be beneficial, but it's important to ensure you are in the low risk category.'

Laura Smith, specialist community public health nurse (health visitor) Ebonie Chandraraj, specialist community public health nurse (health visitor) @gentlehealthvisitors

Supporting your baby's development

LOTS OF NEW parents ask me about specific ways to support their baby's development. Your natural instincts will often serve you best, as we'll come on to, but there are a few things you may want to consider. Once again, a few experts join us to support my advice to you. This section is all about supporting you to get off to a positive start, to build on or begin bonding.

Not all mothers love their baby instantly. Some do, but some don't. It can take time to build a bond and get to know your baby. It's not uncommon for anyone to need time to get to know someone before falling in love. Some mums also say their baby isn't who they expected them to be. A mum once told me she looked at her baby and thought, 'Who are *you* then?' Please don't judge yourself if you don't get that instant rush of love. You might be overwhelmed or exhausted, and these are strong feelings that will likely override feelings of bonding or even love at times. Exhaustion isn't something you can just brush off and replace with love. You need to rest/sleep – it's a need for human survival. Try not to underestimate the importance of your human survival needs in order to flourish as a person and a mother – you need to meet those, mama. Doing very simple things with your baby, like sitting in skin-to-skin or smelling the top of their tiny beautiful head, may also help to build your bond as you learn and grow together.

MUMSTINCT

Biology, physiology and instinct will likely guide you better than I can in this book – never underestimate the power of your maternal instinct . . . 'mumstinct' as I like to call it. The more in tune you are with your body and your true self postnatally, the more likely it is that you'll find your natural intuition takes over and you'll know what to do and how to support your baby. As we've seen, your brain has and continues to undergo changes to support you to care for your baby. Nature is really incredible, and ever so intelligent.

That said, if you have had a difficult birth experience or have a mental health problem, such as PND/anxiety, you may need to address your mental health first before you can feel confident to trust yourself. For mums who do not have any concerns over their mental health, it can still take time to feel in tune with yourself and therefore your instincts. As you go through this transition to become a mother and process what that really means for you, your mumstinct will likely evolve and show up more frequently for you. Your own early child-hood experiences may also impact how you feel about motherhood, and childhood memories may reappear, or you may find yourself making compar-isons. Our own attachment to our parents can play a role in how we parent – it's normal to look back at how we were raised and even start to analyse that a bit. That's the liberating thing about parenthood: we now have the opportunity to make 'the rules', to do what we would have preferred as children or to take the amazing things our parents did for us into our own children's lives. We do have the freedom to decide how we want to manage situations and our approaches. There are many rules in life, a lot of red tape these days and regulations, but not in parenting (I need not state the obvious about when that does not apply).

That said, deciding on how we deal with things motherhood throws at us may not always be easy. Sometimes we are driven by our emotions, and don't know any other way to manage ourselves. We are social and emotional creatures after all. And that's okay – it's part of what makes us human. What I would like to take a moment to think about here is the idea of parenting ourselves before we par-ent our babies/children. It's very difficult for these to be independent, and although I am certainly no parenting guru, I really do understand the importance of looking at ourselves first. The more I have studied my own behaviour and reactions, the more I have come to realise that sometimes my reaction isn't to Georgie's behaviour, but to how I feel about myself or what I want her to do. Babies and toddlers will test you – without even meaning to at times – and, with-out knowing your true self, it can be hard to act in a way you would prefer to. I am all for discussions around how to deal with particular situations and for general parenting advice – there's some great information and accounts out there. But I can't deny that I always come back to looking at how mothers are treated and how we treat ourselves first. It can be very difficult at times for us to follow the advice of experts when we are depleted, feel abandoned, lonely, exhausted and misunderstood. I know that's a lot of negativity right there, but those feelings are real for many mothers, who then go and read a post saying that they can or should be doing better for their kids. What those mums need is what I certainly needed at times too: some authentic self-care, compassion and a moment to look at myself, not my kid. I needed to explore some of my emotions and comfort myself before I was able to really comfort her. Self-care could, at times, be the key to us feeling more able to be the best versions of ourselves. If you have any deep issues related to your own childhood, or anything you feel you want to explore, psychotherapy may be a great option if you have the time and budget for it.

I will put my hand up now and say that postnatal anxiety did not allow me to be guided by my mumstinct and I needed support, but it came a little later on in the journey, after the depths of sleep deprivation and going back to work. If you are experiencing any problems with your emotional wellbeing or mental health, please reach out either to someone close to you or to a healthcare professional (see page 244).

Getting back to supporting your baby's development and bonding, below are some simple things you can do.

BABY MASSAGE

~~~~

This is becoming more popular now in the UK. I did it with Georgie and it was great for the both of us. There are so many benefits to massage, such as encouraging digestion and supporting your baby to create space within their body and stretch out. This stretching can aid sleep, reduce wind and encourage movement – and therefore the passing of wind!

Heading to a baby class can also help with getting out of the home and making local mum friends. We would have a cuppa and a chat afterwards and I really looked forward to that interaction with others going through exactly the same thing. It's powerful. With your first baby, everything is so new – you don't have a routine and are mostly winging it. Clinically, I knew what I was doing because of my midwifery knowledge, but implementing routine and parenting styles was all brand new and overwhelming, so it was extremely helpful to chat things through with other mums.

If you go to a baby massage class, there may be days when your baby isn't up for a massage and stimulation. They may be tired, want to cluster-feed or just lie on you in skin-to-skin. That's okay – all teachers know this and so do the mums next to you. Please don't put any pressure on yourself or your baby to complete the class. If you need to feed or even walk out, try not to worry – you won't upset anyone by doing so. Newborns are unpredictable; there's no such thing as a 'good' baby. Later on we will talk about different personalities and how, by the time your baby is one, you will be able to tell whether they are more introvert or extrovert (see page 186).

Kat King, featured earlier on pages 27, 68 and 69, is a qualified baby massage teacher too. I went to her classes with Georgie and asked her to tell me more about the benefits of baby massage. She said:

'Baby massage has been widely practised in other cultures for many years. In India, baby massage techniques are often handed down from mother to daughter. In Ayurveda, sesame oil would be used, but you can use coconut oil or a specific baby one.

Babies can be massaged from birth. However, we build up the timelines as they grow. Newborn babies will probably only enjoy five minutes of massage.

Benefits of baby massage:

- Encourages muscle coordination and joint flexibility for baby
- Stimulates lymph flow
- Encourages relaxed breathing
- Helps with wind and colic
- Creates the bond between parents and baby
- Helps to calm and relax the parents
- Builds trust and supports communication

For slightly older babies, baby massage works well before or after a bath (be aware that baby will be slippery), ideally on an empty tummy.

Make sure the room is warm and comfortable and place baby on a warm towel.

Remember you are giving baby a soothing, calm, loving touch. It will help you build confidence the more you practise. Joining a baby massage group with a qualified instructor and other parents is a great way to get out and meet new friends.'

Kat King, doula and yoga teacher, Loveuyoga

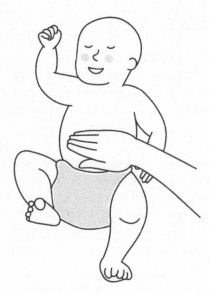

Massage 1: Stomach hold
Brings warmth and encourages
relaxation

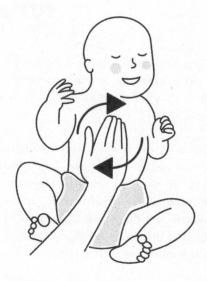

Massage 2: Full circle movement
Pushes food and gas through
the digestive system

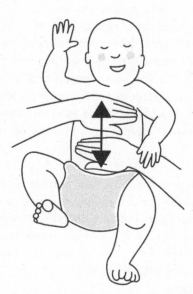

Massage 3: Stomach stroking
Encourages air bubbles down

TUMMY TIME

~~~~

Tummy time is recommended soon after birth for most babies. If your baby needs admission to the neonatal unit, do speak to the specialist team about this. They will be able to explain when it's safe for your baby to have tummy time.

Some mums who have had a vaginal birth and are planning on breastfeeding do tummy time – at birth! This is also known as the breast crawl, where babies are left on their mum's tummy to make their way to the breast. Incredibly, babies will find their way by crawling to the breast unassisted. It's magical to watch and there are clips available online – type in 'newborn baby breast crawl'. It is believed that babies who crawl to the breast at birth and latch themselves on end up with a more efficient latch.

Getting back to tummy time, this helps develop stronger neck and shoulder muscles, improves motor skills, and supports babies to roll over. It's only advisable to put your baby on their tummy when awake and under supervision – see safe sleeping position advice on page 100.

Most babies don't like tummy time, and certainly won't after a feed. You might find they prefer tummy time on a special tummy time pillow you can buy. Always ensure you do not leave them unattended with any products like this, though – not even for a minute. Overall, try not to worry if you don't manage to get them on their tummy for long. Responding to your baby and being guided by them is more important than following recommendations strictly. As you get to know you baby's wake windows you may start to be able to develop a little bit of a routine around it, but there's no pressure to do this. You do what works for you both.

You can start by putting your baby on their tummy, lying them down on your chest or across your lap for about a minute or two at a time. You might have to keep encouraging your baby, building up the time spent on their front, and, eventually, most will get used to it. Georgie, however, wouldn't give in and hated tummy time, even with the bribery of toys. We never met the recommendation of 45 minutes per day by three months, broken into shorter intervals. Maybe you'll have better luck.

SKIN-TO-SKIN

Skin-to-skin really is as simple as it sounds – you literally strip your baby down to their nappy (some parents like to remove the nappy too, if they're feeling brave) and have your bare skin touching your baby's. Touching your baby is one of the most natural desires in the world and you'll likely have an instinctive pull towards physical contact, whether that be in skin-to-skin, touching their cheeks or kissing them.

Researchers have identified many benefits – from better temperature regulation, heart rate and respiratory rate control, reduction in stress responses and crying (babies) to increased oxytocin production, enhanced developmental support, and improved breastfeeding rates and lengths (mums). Skin-to-skin contact has a calming effect on both of you. Combining skin-to-skin with feeding is perfect, for both breast- and bottle-feeding parents. Being in skin-to-skin can also encourage babies that may be a little reluctant to feed initially to take to the breast.

I always advise new parents to have skin-to-skin with their baby for as often and as long as possible and recommend skin-to-skin for all ages. During that first year of life, skin-to-skin is important throughout, if you feel comfortable with it.

THE IMPACT OF SEPARATION

We have known for a while about the heartbreaking impacts and disruption to the family when mums and babies are separated for extended periods. Some of you may find the information I am about to share upsetting, but I decided to write about the terrible impacts mums and babies suffered during the COVID-19 pandemic because I want to raise awareness and ensure those mums feel heard – their anger and pain are valid. I hope that, if we are ever presented with a similar situation, we do the optimal thing for women and their babies: **we keep mothers and their infants together**.

Research by the World Health Organization shows that COVID-19 severely affected the care given to small and sick newborns, resulting in unnecessary suffering and loss. A study published in the *Lancet's eClinicalMedicine* highlights the critical importance of ensuring newborn babies have very close contact with parents after birth, especially for those born small (at low birth weight) or prematurely. However, in many countries, when COVID-19 was confirmed or even suspected, newborn babies were routinely separated from their mums. This separation put them at higher risk of poor outcomes, lifelong health complications and even death. According to the report, disruptions to kangaroo mother care – which involves close contact between a parent, usually a mother, and a newborn baby – will exacerbate these risks.

The Lancet concludes: 'Up to 125,000 babies' lives could be saved with full coverage of kangaroo mother care. For babies born preterm or at low birth weight, kangaroo mother care is particularly critical.' Reading that is painful, I know – those babies and mothers deserved better.

If you and your baby are separated for any reason or you don't feel like doing skin-to-skin, remember that it does not have to be with you. A loving caregiver can provide this bodily support to your baby, achieving the same positive impacts.

WHY BABYWEARING MATTERS

Baby slings or carriers can tick so many boxes for both of you: they enable you to carry your baby around (they're usually happier being with you) and distribute their weight evenly, supporting your arms, shoulders and back, all while keeping you hands-free so you have a bit more leeway to moisturise your face or make a cuppa! Meeting baby's needs and your own at the same time: win-win! They can also be great if you've got any other children, as a sling enables you to carry your baby while doing more with your older child: playing with them, cooking for them, feeding them and generally having a little more freedom.

Zoë from The Sling Consultancy is an expert in baby-carrying and has some great posts on Instagram (@theslingconsultancy) about the science behind babywearing. She kindly shares some of the most important findings below, together with some more generalised advice:

'Slings/carriers can be used safely from birth into toddlerhood and beyond if it is something you find helpful to use. If your baby was born prematurely or is under the weight limit of your sling/carrier, seek support from a trained and insured babywearing consultant as there are always ways to carry safely. These babies often need more contact and support, which helps their growth and development.

Ensuring you are using a sling/carrier as safely as possible is key to reducing the risk of suffocation, which can occur if a carrier/sling is too loose, poorly fitting or not used in line with guidance, so if you do use one be very mindful of your baby's airway and ensure you follow these five safety TICKS steps from the UK Sling Consortium:

1. T is for Tight
2. I is for In View at All Times
3. C is for Close Enough to Kiss
4. K is for Keep Chin Off the Chest
5. S is for Supported Back

As baby develops, typically around three to five months, they may want to have their arms out of the carrier, to be more mobile when awake and to see more as their eyesight develops, so hip carriers can be super helpful and, from around six months, back carrying can make things easier if they are too big on your front. It can also be really helpful when travelling or doing things that aren't feasible or accessible with prams/buggies. There are toddler- and pre-schooler-sized carriers for older ones too. Carrying is simply a useful tool to have as a parent, and the more tools we have at our fingertips the better! It doesn't make you a certain 'type' of parent, it doesn't mean they won't walk eventually; it means you have something to help when they don't want to walk or they are tired.

There are so many slings/carriers on the market these days and just because it is a well-known brand or is expensive doesn't mean it is going to work for you and your child. It can be helpful to try a few on to see what you like or don't like. If something isn't working or you are finding it uncomfortable, do seek support. You may have a local sling library or consultant, or many will do sessions online, or consultants may have free-to-access resources such as blogs or YouTube videos [see page 241].'

Zoë, babywearing educational consultant, The Sling Consultancy

Georgie lived in a sling for several months after birth and we both loved it. I used to pop her in the sling and go off for a walk, listen to a podcast and grab myself a coffee (being mindful of hot liquids over her head). I miss those days, as hard as they were – enjoy it while you can pop them in there and get on with your bits and bobs! At the next developmental phase, containing them safely in one area can be a full-blown operation (we cover that on pages 210–11 and I've got a little list to help with safety when the time comes).

EYE CONTACT, TALKING AND SINGING

At birth, your baby recognises your voice and your smell. Spending time talking, singing or playing music (for you both) can be a good way of reminding your baby they're safe in the new world they have been born into. Even if it does seem alien to them, they still have some home comforts they remember from the time they spent inside your body. And many rituals, singing, prayers, dancing and even common greeting behaviours all seem to follow patterns and rhythms, providing comfort and stress reduction. Anthropologists too have written about the anxiety-reducing effects of singing, praying or crying together. These behaviours often occurred in tribes when faced with disasters or traumas such as epidemics and famine, or when preparing for war. Many scientists believe the positive psychological effects of music on mood are likely linked to the rhythm in music.

As you have possibly experienced first-hand, rocking, patting or singing is an instinctive behaviour we quickly draw upon when soothing a baby. Or even an adult, if you think about it – when soothing a crying adult we will often rub their back or shoulder in a rhythmic action. In children, rhythmical behaviours such as leg swinging are also associated with a decrease in heart rate. Singing in particular has been proven to reduce stress and even enhance cognitive development. Two Harvard Medical School researchers found that singing lullabies to infants helped to soothe and calm them when crying or distressed. When directing a song at your baby, you're communicating more than just the song – you're letting them know they're safe, you're close by and they have your attention, all of which is very reassuring for babies. Singing also helps older babies with memory, language and communication.

It can take some weeks before your baby makes conscious eye contact with you. At birth they can only see as far as 8–15 inches, so get up nice and close when you're attempting to make eye contact. By 12 weeks you may get a genuine (toothless) smile – the amount of joy this can bring parents is possibly one of the most beautiful parts of parenthood. How is it possible to love this little person so much so quickly? What a privilege it is to be a part of.

BABY SIGNING

Teaching babies to sign as a way of communicating before learning speech is becoming very popular, for good reason. It's a lovely way to spend time and bond with your baby, and also to meet other parents. Some parents really value being able to communicate with their babies at such a young age; from four months a baby may be able to start to recognise signs and by nine months those who attend regular classes may be able to sign back!

However, some claims about the benefits may not be supported by hard evidence. Although initially babies who learn to sign may be better communicators, researchers found that when babies were 30 months and 36 months old there was no statistically significant difference between groups. Simply put, there is no evidence at present that babies benefit in a lasting way. Overall, though, I think it's a lovely idea and something you may want to look into doing, but avoid being guided by some claims of higher IQs – they're not founded on evidence, so don't feel any pressure to get to a class.

PLAY AND MOVEMENT

In the first few months of life babies are exploring and linking sight of their hands and arms to the feeling of movement and the impact they can have on their environment. They don't play as such – their little life is mostly about adjusting to life outside the womb, listening and moving. Newborn babies are capable of making conscious movement and this has been proven when studied.

Walking in a forest, lying on a blanket watching the clouds, and moving around with your baby are all experiences that support brain development – and the more varied the better. Another reason why babywearing (see pages 112–14) can be such a great way of supporting your baby's development.

YOUR BABY'S TEMPERAMENT

All babies are born with different temperaments and, by the end of the fourth trimester, it's likely you'll know a little bit about your baby's personality. Some are quieter than others, less fazed by their new environment and adapting to life outside the womb, while others find it a little more difficult. Remember the difference between the babies on pages 61 and 63?

If this is your first baby, you may find it takes a little more time to get to know them. If this isn't your first baby, you'll see the difference and be able to compare – making it a bit easier. Siblings are usually very different, too, even when they have a similar upbringing.

HONESTY BOX

From birth, Georgie was (and I hate to label her but I must be honest) a very high-need baby. She needed me a lot – to be on me, to feel comforted and to be stimulated when she was up for it. She was not one of those babies who would lie content, looking around and listening. She was also absolutely disgusted when I tried to give her a dummy before a nap once. How dare I offer her anything other than my boob? It's funny to look back on, as she still has very strong opinions on what she will and won't accept – and I admire her for that. The baby I met at birth is the little person I now know.

Crying

ALL BABIES CRY to varying degrees because they are genetically pro-grammed to do so. They need to be able to alert you to what it is they need and, as you know, crying is their only form of communication for some time. Even as they get older and are better able to express themselves, crying, or making irritable sounds, is still one of the first things they revert to. Crying can be a healthy release, even for adults.

CRYING AND HUMAN RITUALS

There is a fascinating piece of research into adult rituals, comforting behaviours and infant crying that I recently read up on. In summary it highlights how there are several calming effects of certain yoga mantras and prayers, as they all possess similar rhythmical attributes to crying. When you think about it (unless they're hurt) a baby's crying bout typically starts with irregular sound patterns. Then, if this fails, the baby will progress to the next phase of crying, which is more rhythmical and there is less variation in spacing between the crying sounds made. Phase two, if we can refer to it as that, follows a predictable pattern. It's this phase of crying which is more of an attempt to self-soothe. Different cries serve different purposes. Phase one is 'Alert caregiver', phase two is 'Caregiver hasn't come or relieved me – self-soothe through the rhythm of crying while continuing to alert caregiver'.

Although we've all heard a baby cry at some point, I hadn't considered the rhythm of it and how that affects the baby's brain or the attempt to self-soothe until I looked into the research about differences in cries and their purpose.

COMMON REASONS FOR CRYING

Now we know a bit more about crying, let's cover the most common causes. You'll know most of these, but I've summarised here so you have a little list to hand.

Hunger

This is one of the most common reasons young babies cry. Their brains aren't quite developed enough to anticipate hunger so, by the time they realise they're hungry and need a feed, a message is sent directly to the brain, alerting the baby to alert you (or whoever is caring for them) that they need to be fed. This can happen pretty quickly, causing a quick escalation which may catch you out. Despite knowing this, Georgie did catch me out a couple of times. Babies may also display hunger signs when they're in need of comfort, as sucking releases feel-good hormones. Sometimes it can be difficult to tell the difference. As babies grow, and once feeding is established, they naturally regulate their feeds and have longer gaps in between, which may help you to prepare.

Wet or dirty nappy

Some babies don't mind a dirty nappy and others cry right away. You'll soon find out whether your baby is bothered by this or not.

Tiredness

Babies do not have the neurological capacity to self-regulate. When we are tired, we recognise this feeling (often during parenthood!). We have a strong coffee, nap if we can, or factor it into our day and slow down if possible. Your baby has no idea – they just feel the discomfort of tiredness. Try to look out for signs, such as yawning, rubbing eyes and disengaging eye contact, and becoming restless, and support them to sleep where possible. You can do this by quietening things down – *shhh* – or reducing/blocking out the light.

When they're really tiny, babies will tend to sleep anywhere, but as they get closer to coming out of the fourth trimester, they may find it a little more difficult. When a baby becomes overtired, they find it hard to calm down again, which can cause you to feel anxious and, in turn, the baby picks up on this and is even less likely to settle. A change of environment or person can help. We have battled overtiredness a lot with Georgie. It took me a while to adjust to her individual sleep needs. Don't worry, you'll get there; just try to observe your baby's behaviour and react as soon as you see those sleepy cues.

Pain

This is usually a different kind of cry to the above-mentioned, and tends to be high-pitched and sudden in onset. Or your baby may show other signs they're in pain, such as drawing up their knees or appearing frustrated/red-faced. If you think your baby's crying because they're in pain then check them over thoroughly – take their temperature, strip them down and have a look at their body. If this persists, give your midwife or health visitor a call. If you have any serious concerns over your baby, you can always take them to A&E. Trust your instincts here.

SIGNS OF SEPSIS

Sepsis – overwhelming infection – is rare, but it can be life-threatening so it's important that we look at the signs and symptoms. Once again, though, I'd like to remind you how important your judgement as a mum is.

The most common and concerning signs are:

- Pale, blue, blotchy skin
- Fast breathing
- Rash that doesn't fade with pressure from a glass
- High-pitched cry
- Weak and very sleepy
- Reluctant to feed
- Temperature of 38°C or more

If your baby has any of these symptoms, take them to A&E straight away or call an ambulance depending on how unwell they appear.

Overstimulation

This can be as hard to deal with as boredom. Babies' brains are like sponges, but can only take so much at a time. An overstimulated baby will often become fretful and be difficult to settle, which may be mistaken for many other things. If your baby appears to be fretful and doesn't settle with rocking or cuddling, try taking them into a quiet, low-lit room and just hold them or stroke their little head and gently *shh-shh* and calmly talk to them. It may take a little while to settle them, but stick with it unless they become increasingly distressed.

Wanting a cuddle

Babies have emotional needs and, having spent nine months tucked up in a nice cosy womb feeling secure, they can often feel a little lost when out in the big wide world. Cuddling and carrying babies is important for their emotional development and growing ability to self-regulate. So you don't need to hold back from cuddling your baby or picking them up. It will not make them clingy; in fact, it will help them become more independent. When you're tired or 'touched out', it's always okay to hand your baby over to another loving caregiver to give yourself a break. Holding or carrying a baby all day is tiring! If you're alone, remember your sling and how that may help you get around while keeping your baby happy too (see pages 112–14).

Being too hot or too cold

Babies have immature temperature regulation which means parents have to regulate it for them. Babies lose heat from their heads so these should be left uncovered at all times when in the home. If a baby looks flushed it may be that they are too hot. Start by taking a layer off them. You may need to check their temperature to see if they are hot due to a fever. Equally, babies may alert you to being cold by crying. A great way to help them regulate their temperature is to have skin-to-skin contact.

TOP TIPS FOR DUMMY USAGE

It's up to you whether you would like to use a dummy or not. Some mums love them, some don't like the idea. Like everything, dummies have their pros and cons. For example, they can increase the risk of infections (particularly middle ear) but they may also be a great way of soothing your baby and aiding sleep. Some research suggests they may reduce the risk of SIDS. If I'm honest, I am not entirely convinced by this and would need to see more research to confidently tell you that is the case. As always, you do you!

- If you choose to use a dummy and are breastfeeding, it's best to wait until the feeding is well established.
- Use the dummy when your baby goes to sleep and avoid using during awake time.
- It's a good idea to stop using a dummy before going to sleep between 6 and 12 months.

- Gently offer your baby the dummy and avoid putting it back in if your baby spits it out – like Georgie did!
- Don't use a neck cord.
- Although common practice back in the day, avoid putting anything on the dummy – such as alcohol.
- Opt for an orthodontic dummy because it adapts to your baby's mouth shape.

COLIC

Studies have shown that approximately 20 per cent of infants cry for long periods without any apparent reason during the first four months. On average, they'll cry for two to three hours a day and this usually reaches a peak at around six weeks. If this happens, of course explore all the potential reasons, but please don't doubt yourself or your ability and do make sure you ask for help. Hearing your baby cry for prolonged periods of time can be deeply distressing. I've shared some of my own experience in the honesty box below. Again, if you need a break and have someone available to hand over to, take the opportunity when you feel the need and try not to be the only one offering comfort. Sometimes a change of energy can help to soothe a baby, so there's no need to feel bad about that.

There are also several remedies available. I'd always suggest you have a chat with your midwife or health visitor before giving your young baby any medication or remedy, just so they can support you with guidance on recommendations and ensure your baby is checked over appropriately. This can be such a stressful time anyway; it's a good idea to offload and get real-life reassurance – if nothing else. Áine, also known as 'The Baby Reflux Lady', is mentioned later on (see pages 123–4), and she can be a great source of support and shares a lot of information about colic online.

Causes of colic are often unknown; however, guidelines from the National Institute for Health and Care Excellence (NICE) and the NHS Choices website both suggest that some babies may have short-term problems with digesting lactose (a natural milk sugar found in breast and formula milk). This is called 'transient lactase deficiency'. Other experts say colic is not a condition but a symptom of the adjustment to life outside the womb, an immature digestive system, gas, silent reflux, and exposure to different bodily sensations.

HONESTY BOX

Georgie was a very quiet baby for about four weeks – she was 2.6kg (5lb 7oz) at birth and three weeks before her due date, as mentioned. It took her four weeks to fully arrive into the world and respond to her new environment. At around five weeks of age she got more vocal, and from around seven to nine weeks she screamed for hours in the evening. Every. Single. Night. It was very upsetting and terribly stressful. I clearly remember dreading 6pm as I knew she would be inconsolable. Andy and I had to mentally prepare for it. We tried everything: swaddling, skin-to-skin, baby massage, swaying, rocking, cradling, carrying, walking, sitting in darkness, playing white noise, playing music we'd listened to during pregnancy, and singing. I even reduced the huge amount of spicy food I ate! Nothing worked.

There are many opinions on the cause of colic. Many experts believe that extended crying may be due to immaturity of the gut and digestion, in particular the fact they do not produce enough amylase – the enzyme required to break down carbohydrates.

One night, Georgie didn't cry at 6pm and I was over the moon – I thought that was it (as colic usually self-resolves and settles eventually). But by 10pm she was screaming more than ever. By midnight I was beyond exhausted and beside myself, so I handed her (and the baby carrier) over to Andy and asked him to take her for a walk. I could hear her screaming down the street – my poor neighbours – and I was in the fetal position in bed, so tired but unable to sleep. A few days later it did self-resolve and we were left with scream-free, peaceful evenings. Finally, we were able to enjoy time as a family again. She still has a bit of a funny turn at 6pm every evening – a rush of energy and a run around. Some experts believe this is due to being overtired, but others say it's a case of them releasing the day's last burst of energy, ready to relax overnight.

REFLUX

Reflux is very common – around 50 per cent of babies in the UK are reported to experience some sort of reflux – and it can leave parents feeling distressed.

I spoke to a lovely paediatrician I know, Dr Richard Daniels, and have summarised his thoughts below.

Reflux is usually caused by a combination of factors. Babies spend a lot of time lying down, so gravity does not help keep milk in their stomachs. Milk is also less viscous than solid food so will run back up the food pipe more easily. The food pipe itself is shorter, which means that there is less distance for the refluxate to travel before it causes symptoms. Some of these can include fussing around feed time, bringing up milk, discomfort or crying after feeds or when lying on their backs. Most children grow out of reflux as they get older.

Within the medical world there are two approaches to managing reflux: lifestyle changes and medication. Lifestyle changes include things like giving smaller feeds more often to reduce the amount of milk in the stomach that can reflux up into the food pipe, and keeping a child upright for a period after feeding to allow gravity to assist while the stomach empties.

'The medication approach is less successful. In most cases, it is just a smaller dose of a medication used for adults with acid reflux, but the cause of their symptoms is different and so the action of these medications is not targeted at the root cause. Infant Gaviscon can help, however, as it sits on top of the stomach contents and so refluxes up the food pipe first, which is less irritating and causes fewer symptoms.

Remember, this gets better with age and, while it can be distressing, it does not cause any long-term problems, especially if baby is putting weight on appropriately.'

Dr Richard Daniels

As a midwife, I have referred many parents to a paediatrician or specialist for advice and support. I spoke to Áine Homer, a.k.a. The Baby Reflux Lady, who is a leading expert on the holistic management and resolution of reflux in babies.

She believes that we should reframe reflux as a symptom rather than a disease in its own right, and stop normalising something simply because it is common. With this new viewpoint on baby reflux, silent reflux and colic, we start to ask why is baby so uncomfortable in their own body and this allows us to take very specific actions to support them and their physical comfort. She has written a very interesting book on the topic, *The Baby Reflux Lady's Survival Guide*. Here's what she advised:

'Firstly, parents should know they're not alone. They might feel like they're alone, they might feel like nobody understands, and they might feel like they're not heard or being listened to. This, combined with the sleep deprivation and being told that reflux is normal, can have a huge impact on their mental health, confidence in parenting and the feelings of isolation, especially if those around them appear to have everything in hand.

There is a silent stigma attached to having a baby with reflux, because those who have not experienced it cannot comprehend the levels of stress it introduces into a new or growing family.

With the normalisation of reflux, many parents end up feeling like it must be their fault that their baby is crying so much. **Reflux is never a parent's fault**.

It may help for parents to understand the different medical terms used to diagnose what is going on. Gastro oesophageal reflux (GOR) is the proper name for reflux that happens from the stomach. Silent reflux is when the regurgitate does not come out of baby's mouth, instead it comes up the throat, perhaps into the mouth or back of the nasal passages. Gastro oesophageal reflux disease (GORD) is simply when the regurgitation "causes marked distress". All of these terms are summarised under "reflux".

Simply put, reflux is regurgitation – the movement of stomach contents into the oesophagus (food pipe). The bodily functions of burping, hiccupping and vomiting mean that the ability to regurgitate is completely normal. What is not normal in infants is the frequency with which it occurs, and the discomfort and pain associated with it.

There is always a cause of reflux. Over the last 10 years I have documented over 30 different things that can cause or contribute to reflux in babies. This is why there is no one-size-fits-all answer, and adult reflux and infantile reflux are completely different, although commonly compared!

Every baby is telling us what is going on for them with their symptoms and behaviours, and our job is to be Sherlock Holmes and piece them together. I advise parents what to observe, such as events during pregnancy, birth and baby's feeding and sleeping patterns and behaviours, digestive symptoms and more. Then we put these observations together like a jigsaw, so that they can see the whole picture. This then informs parents what actions to take to support their baby's comfort.

Regardless of what is going on for any baby, the holistic approach of understanding all their symptoms and behaviours first can be hugely insightful for parents.'

Áine Homer, holistic baby reflux specialist

It's worth exploring all options with your paediatric team and you may also consider reaching out to a specialist like Áine if your baby does suffer with reflux.

JAUNDICE

The transition to extrauterine life is extraordinary. The fetal circulatory system is one of the most remarkable on earth: oxygenated blood flows through veins and deoxygenated blood flows through arteries, yet, once born, there are special shunts in the heart that close shortly after birth and redirect blood to switch this system around. Oxygenated blood then flows through arteries and deoxygenated blood flows through veins. To look at a baby at birth you would never know the complex transition the body effortlessly makes to adapt to life outside the womb, and this is something that will always fascinate me.

Jaundice is usually a normal physiological process that most babies go through as part of another adaption. As we know, life in the womb is very different and babies need more red blood cells to grow, keep them well oxygenated and protect them at birth. Once born, babies need to adjust themselves for oxygenated life via their lungs, and red blood cells are no longer required in the same volume as in the womb. These red blood cells therefore need to be broken down. Around 60 per cent of babies become jaundiced within the first week of life; it rarely starts before 24 hours and usually self-resolves in ten days.

Babies have an immature liver and sometimes struggle to break down red blood cells. One of the by-products is bilirubin, causing jaundice and that yellow appearance of the skin and eyes. Your midwife and health visitor will be checking for jaundice and ensuring they are happy with baby's colour and behaviour, and the amount of wet and dirty nappies they have. *Generally* speaking, a baby who is very alert, waking for feeds, has lots of wet and dirty nappies and is feeding well will not need treatment for jaundice, but on some occasions even these babies will. If you have any concerns over the colour of your baby or their behaviour, call your midwife, health visitor or doctor so that they can appropriately assess your baby. Sometimes babies will need light therapy (phototherapy) – treatment with a special blue light in a cot or incubator – and, in very extreme cases of jaundice, a baby may need a blood transfusion.

HONESTY BOX

Georgie needed treatment for jaundice in hospital with phototherapy. After a blissful home birth, we were separated from Andy due to COVID-19 restrictions. Many mothers experienced the same thing and, although it wasn't for long, around 36 hours in total, being separated was heartbreaking. He wasn't even allowed to drop extra clothes for us to the door. We were on day five, my milk had just come in, baby blues hit (pretty hard) and I was in a side room on my own, sobbing my heart out. One of the healthcare assistants heard me crying from outside the room and came in to check on me. I assured her I was fine, but I think she was concerned about my mental state. I was too, but chose to wipe away the tears and pass it off as just a moment – like a lot of mums do. It wasn't just a moment – I felt awful. I just wanted to get out and back home with my family.

At one point, it was recommended I top Georgie up with either expressed breast milk or formula to help flush out the bilirubin. I chose not to take this advice because I did not want to interfere with our breastfeeding journey. Georgie was feeding like a dream, I had large quantities of milk and she had lots of wet and dirty nappies. After 24 hours of phototherapy, regular feeds and normal blood results, we were ecstatic to be discharged home and reunited with Daddy – without giving her a bottle. A couple of days felt like a lifetime, but once home the baby blues melted away and the tears stopped.

Getting set up at home

THERE ARE MANY items you can buy yourself and your baby these days — there's a product for just about everything. Some are genius inventions; others not so much. You only need to take to social media to see the memes about the difference when leaving home in labour with your first, second and any other babies. You gradually bring less and less, and tend to relax more and more. Not always, though!

If you have already got a little one, you'll likely be set up with lots of the equipment and bits and bobs you need; you've been through the trial and error of it all. If not, you may want to consider creating little stations at home like the ones I've outlined below:

- **Changing station:** an area set up just for changing your baby. It may be a table that comes with fixed compartments or sometimes an inbuilt bath. Another cheaper option is an organiser and mat by the sofa with all the changing bits you need in one place. There's nothing more annoying than having a poo explosion and nothing right near you. You may also want two changing stations: one in your bedroom and one in your lounge area, for example. Try to keep these topped up or delegate someone else to do it, if that is an option for you.
- **Feeding station:** similar to the changing station, this is just for you or whoever is feeding your baby. Set yourself up in two areas where you're regularly feeding your baby; ensure you're as comfortable as possible, maybe with your feeding pillows and/or back/neck support. Leave water bottles and a snack box there. I had a little wooden box I picked up from a pound shop and popped some fruit, healthy bars, cartons of juice and dark choc in there.
- **Sleeping arrangements and safe sleeping plan:** see page 101 for more info from The Lullaby Trust on safe sleeping.

KEY POINTS

- The fourth trimester is about healing, adjusting and adapting. Go easy on yourself.
- Avoid postnatal depletion by eating nutrient-dense, easily digestible food, resting, incorporating gentle movement when you're up to it and *asking for help*.
- Try not to let the pressures of the Western world creep into your life at this time. Remember what our ancestors and many countries around the world have in common: honour those first 42 days.
- Report any pain or concerns as soon as possible, particularly around wounds: infection delays recovery.
- All babies cry; there's no such thing as a 'good' baby. They all have high needs, require regular feeding and want to be cuddled or held a lot.
- You'll never get back those precious moments with your baby. Ignore whatever or whoever is less important. Try to stay present in the moment and move on when you want to.
- Try not to let the external world pop your newborn bubble. Remain in control of who deserves your attention at this time.
- You're doing amazing, I promise.

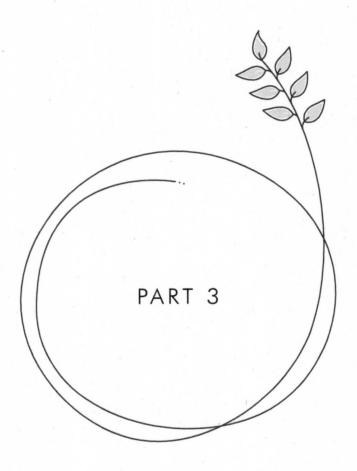

PART 3

Three to Six Months

As we covered in the previous section, throughout the fourth trimester you're recovering from birth, adjusting to life with a new baby, establishing breast-feeding or getting to grips with bottle-feeding, and dealing with sleep deprivation and any newborn conditions, such as colic. Coming out of the fourth trimester is another milestone for both of you. A lot happens between three and six months – from a huge developmental leap and signs of teething to changes in sleep needs – and we'll cover all that in this section. We'll also discuss how you can support your baby and find out why they aren't passively allowing the world to go by and instead are constantly actively seeking out things to compare and learning about the environment around them.

As always, I'm going to be very honest with you about my personal experi-ences, offer some ideas about what you can expect to see from your baby and share some expert advice. We will start off with the lighter topics and get to the deeper issues a bit later on in this section.

Lastly, although we'll cover a lot about your baby's brain and how to support them to develop, remember that your brain is also developing as a parent. Your brain changed during pregnancy and continues to change postnatally; it corresponds with your baby's. Parenting is not something you are just ready to 'do' – it involves a lot of learning as you get to know your baby and as your brains experience synchronicity. Go easy on yourself. You're doing an amaz-ing job – no one on the planet is born a perfect parent, I can promise you that. We are all learning on the job and that's okay. No matter what you see on social media, we all have our struggles.

What to expect

ALL BABIES ARE different and do things at different times. Following your child's inner timeline is important for the development of their self-esteem and self-worth because it is sending them a message that *their* timeline is okay. There is a lot out there about developmental milestones and you'll often notice quite a variation in times given for certain things. For example, walking is 'normal' from ten to 18 months – an entire eight-month window of normality . . . that's a big window and reflects the fact that there's no real specific time. So try not to compare your baby with your friends' babies – it's perfectly normal for them all to do things at different paces and isn't a reflection on you as a mum. Some parents find this harder than expected and become a little fixated on what their babies are doing, or not doing, yet.

Feeling a little uptight about timelines is very common and totally understandable. We all want the best for our babies, for them to meet their milestones and provide visible confirmation that they are healthy and well. Where possible, try to be led by your baby's pace, praising or gently encouraging them but not forcing. They will get there in their own time.

From 16 weeks onwards, you may see your baby:

- sit up with support
- choose specific objects to pick up and bring to their mouths
- push themselves up, using their hands and arms, usually during tummy time
- look around more consciously/become more aware
- babble, gurgle, make sounds and try to copy sounds
- roll over
- show signs of teething (dribbling, biting and appearing to be in discomfort)
- start to recognise signs (such as the milk sign!), if you are signing

If you don't see these milestones appearing right away, please, as I mentioned above, try not to worry. If you do have concerns, please always speak to your health visitor as they will be able to assess your baby and provide you with reassurance or any further advice/support you need.

AN ATTACHMENT TO YOU

Your baby will generally prefer to be with the person they have spent most time with and that's usually (but not always) Mum. Your smell, voice and touch are a familiar comfort to them. Attachment and dependency are different things. Coming out of the fourth trimester, your baby may not seem quite so dependent on you, but the attachment to you will likely grow stronger. Around this age they may also become vocal about wanting you and start crying in the arms of other people – even family members they know, but especially people they do not know very well. This is very natural and normal behaviour and does not mean you have a clingy baby. Instead, it means you have built a strong bond and trust. Your baby has emotional ties to a familiar face versus an unfamiliar face. It's very important for them to know what they can trust and who they are safe with.

SMILING AND GIGGLES

Around this age, your baby will become more aware and interactive and you will get some genuine smiles, if not already, and giggles. Their first little laugh emerging around this age is usually the biggest highlight of motherhood so far. Your ability to communicate grows – and what a beautiful thing that is. For the next few months, your baby will be working on their social skills and the smiles will often start to extend to others, although not all babies smile back just because they can, especially at strangers. Some are more intrigued and interested in examining faces/clothing and their little personality will start to shine through. Just like adults, some babies are more sociable than others. The initial period of poorer vision within the first six months could be due to the need to take in the overall structure of faces rather than being dependent on details. Blurred vision enables babies to cut out all the distractions and is possibly nature's way of getting us to focus on what is important.

TRYING TO COMMUNICATE WITH YOU

At around four to six months your baby will start making noises, babbling and trying to communicate with you. They may even imitate words and noises. Whatever expressions and noises they make, mirroring these is a great way to encourage them and let them know that they're doing well and learning as they should be. It reaffirms their thoughts on how they're moving their face and what they sound like. Research shows that mirroring supports bonding and attachment, but also aids development. Another way they communicate well is via their eye movement. By four months they have good control over their eye movement and can tell you either 'I'm interested in that' or 'That's boring me now'. Babies will stare at things if they're interested in them and look away after a few seconds when they are not. Observing their eye movement will give you a good indication of what it is they find most interesting.

RESPONDING

Babies will also start to respond to noises and sounds as they become familiar with these patterns; for example, your phone ringing or the front door opening. They are always looking for cues and patterns and are hardwired to find these in order to make sense of the world. Identifying facial expressions and associations is an important part of the development of social skills and reading body language. We take for granted how much we subconsciously pick up about others; we're keenly attuned to micro changes in body language and facial expressions, which helps us to recognise when something doesn't 'feel' right. One example is when a person says something that doesn't match their facial expression. Have you ever seen someone smile, but their eyes tell a very different story and looking at them makes you feel uncomfortable?

This skill set of interpreting different facial cues is being built from birth, which is just one of the reasons it's really beneficial for your baby to watch you – technology-free. As I'm writing this, I become aware of my blank expression. You can't read much at all from me right now and that's often how we look while scrolling, reading or messaging. This is definitely worth considering when you're around your baby at this age and they are trying to interpret your facial cues and build on their knowledge of human behaviour and appropriate reactions to the world around them. I know it's really hard to put technology down, to ignore a message or not reply to an email, but building in technology-free time can be a helpful solution. I now set restrictions on myself and shut my apps down or set time limits so that I use my phone wisely and only at certain times.

Babies are learning to become specialised in what is important in their own environment. When babies hear human voices, within about 100 milliseconds there's a flood of electrical activity and they will turn towards the source of those voices. By six months, babies are very good at being able to determine sounds made by all languages around the globe. Babies have the ability to learn any language they want to speak *without* their native accent. Yet learning a language in adulthood almost always results in speaking with an accent from the mother tongue.

HONESTY BOX

I miss Georgie's smell and tiny body so much and am teary as I reminisce about this. You'll never regret having those moments with your baby over replying to a text message or scrolling through social media. Many of us fall victim to feeling the need to reply instantly or keep up with the fast pace of the digital world, but when you take the time to simply be with your baby you hold those memories forever. No one can take them away – they're your preciousness to keep forever. People can, however, take your time, energy and attention away very easily. Remember, you are in control of that, so, when you're with your baby, never feel external pressure to give up your attention for something that's less important to you. Feel free to tell someone interrupting your interaction to 'hang on', or simply ignore them and address your baby first.

MOBILITY

You'll notice that your baby is becoming more mobile and trying to rock from side to side when lying on their back or tummy. This rocking movement is preparation for when they roll over. You might find that this goes on for a while and, as your baby gets stronger, they will probably surprise you by rolling over suddenly, when you are least expecting it! Because of this, you'll need to be more careful where you place your baby, as it's not uncommon for babies to roll off surfaces like beds or changing mats, especially when you turn your back – even for a second. Never leave your baby unattended on a raised surface for that reason.

GROWTH SPURT

It's usual for your baby to have a growth spurt at around 16 weeks. It is very common for babies to be extra hungry and fussy around this time. The evenings can be particularly demanding, especially if you are breastfeeding. This is when breastfeeding mums sometimes decide to introduce an evening/bedtime bottle, or dream feed, to help baby settle. There's no hard and fast rule here – you know what's best for your baby, so follow your instincts or seek professional advice if you're not sure.

IMPROVED MOTOR SKILLS

Babies are born with hundreds of muscles and have no idea how to control them. During the first year of life, a baby will learn more motor skills than at any other time. Between three and six months there's a real acceleration.

'Motor skills' refers to skills related to moving and coordinating muscles. There are two main types: gross and fine motor skills. The gross motor skills involve using the larger muscles in the body; for example, for balance, coordination and physical strength. Fine motor skills include control and precision movement of the small muscles of the hand; for example, grasping and shaking a toy (and, later, using a fork or spoon). Earlier, your baby would grasp using a reflex action and wouldn't be able to let go at will. Now, they should be able to grasp your finger purposely and to release it at will (see pages 178–9 for more on this).

According to Dr Kang Lee at the Dr. Erick Jackman Institute of Child Study, University of Toronto: 'The learning that takes place in the first six months of a child's life forms the foundation from which the child eventually becomes a functioning social being in their society. My advice to parents is that they expose their babies to as wide of an environment as possible, in terms of faces, languages, smells and tastes. This all helps a child live and learn in a globalised world.'

Encouraging your baby to hold age-appropriate toys and introducing them to different environments outside their home can help with this exposure. One idea for this is to take them outside to let them touch the leaves or plants with their little fingers and feel the wind on their face. Another is to take them for a train ride, or for a coffee with your friend, and have them out of the pram; if you have them on your lap or forward-facing in a carrier, they can see and interact with what's going on around them. You don't have to go over the top all in one day – it's the little things you introduce them to throughout the weeks and months that can help. And if you've had a stimulating morning, never feel bad about having a relaxing afternoon with them. You'll naturally expose them to a range of environments, smells, sounds and faces.

What's happening with your baby

BETWEEN THREE AND six months your baby goes through one of their biggest developmental leaps and experiences immense changes, both physically and mentally. Probably the best words to describe the next period are 'more mobile and stronger'. Coming out of the fourth trimester, they go from being fairly vulnerable and unable to hold themselves up to being sturdier, able to move more consciously, and far better able to communicate by six months. For us adults, learning is a conscious decision: we choose the topic and sit down to study or research it. Babies just have to open their eyes – they're learning all the time.

BRAIN-TO-BRAIN SYNCHRONY

It wasn't until the 1970s that parenting studies began in earnest, and only very recently have scientists really been able to see what happens in the brain when parents and babies interact. Traditionally, parent and baby brains were studied separately, but there is an interesting emerging field of neuroscience looking at synchronicity between parent and baby.

Professor Rebecca Saxe, a cognitive neuroscientist from the United States, was one of the first scientists in human history to undertake an MRI scan on a nine-week-old baby – her son Arthur – and then again on her second baby, Percy, aged three months at the time. Incredibly, the scans showed that some areas of a baby's brain already have the same function as they do in adulthood. Babies are particularly interested in faces and facial expressions. Saxe's curious experimentation and drive to discover what babies know led to arguably one of the most interesting findings about such young babies. She found there was a response in the middle frontal lobe when watching human faces on a film shown in the MRI. This area of the brain is specialised in seeing and understanding other people. It is therefore possible that there is a predisposition to who babies learn from, and what they learn, already structured into the anatomy of the brain. In adults that middle frontal lobe region is more active when we are thinking about something we care about, something more valuable or relevant to us. If that area is visibly active on an MRI scan in young babies, I am left wondering whether babies are identifying what is relevant to them and understanding how important that is for them – as a human.

Research has also proved something most of us may have guessed: that multi-sensory stimulation supports healthy brain development in babies. What we may not have been able to guess is how similar a mother's brain's response to this interaction is to that of the baby. You can see certain areas of the brain literally light up simultaneously in both mother and baby. Your voice, touching, and smiling at your baby are very simple, natural and instinctive ways to bond. Emotional connection is critical to baby brain development and their overall wellbeing. Every little stroke, smile and noise you make has an impact over time. By exposing your baby to other sensory stimulation, such as the feel of the wind, the smell of freshly cut grass and the sound of water, you're doing a great job of helping them learn about the world through their senses, which is an integral part of being human. You don't need to do anything extravagant.

CONNECTING WITH YOUR BABY AND THE POWER OF MIRROR NEURONS

The capabilities of the human brain are truly remarkable and I want to highlight the power of mirroring when communicating with your baby. Mirror neurons play a huge role in our ability to understand the world, predict things and empathise. These neurons also make it possible for us to recognise and imitate facial expressions, spread laughter, but also cry while watching a sad movie.

Our ability to simulate situations and imitate behaviours is fundamental to our existence as humans. This is one of the reasons babies love it when you mirror them and why they imitate you. They feel connected to you. These moments, minutes or even seconds of interaction, showing love and being responsive to your baby, may not seem like much, but they are huge and you're doing an incredible job of raising the future.

A lot is going on in the brain when you and your baby are just looking at each other and interacting. We underestimate the power of these little regular interactions – they literally build a brain.

MORE THAN JUST A RED BOOK

If you are concerned about your baby's development, speak to your health visitor and/or GP to discuss any worries you have, even if it's just for peace of mind. You also have the 'red book' (Personal Child Health Record or PCHR) to refer to as that keeps a record of your baby's weight and height and development reviews during the first two years. There's a lot of information in the red book too, with advice and data. Sometimes parents add their own notes, such as details about medication or anything they want to remember.

TEETHING

Until I had Georgie, I didn't know that teething would start from four months, and earlier for some, and continue (on and off) for up to thirty-three months. I was under the impression that teething was a time when most of the teeth come through together within a few months or so, but it does not happen in that way. I wish someone had told me!

Here's a rough guide from the NHS to how babies' teeth usually emerge:

- bottom incisors (bottom front teeth) – these are usually the first to come through, usually at around 5–7 months
- top incisors (top front teeth) – these tend to come through at about 6–8 months
- top lateral incisors (either side of the top front teeth) – these come through at around 9–11 months
- bottom lateral incisors (either side of the bottom front teeth) – these come through at around 10–12 months
- first molars (back teeth) – these come through at around 12–16 months
- canines (between the lateral incisors and the first molars) – these come through at around 16–20 months
- second molars – these come through at around 20–30 months

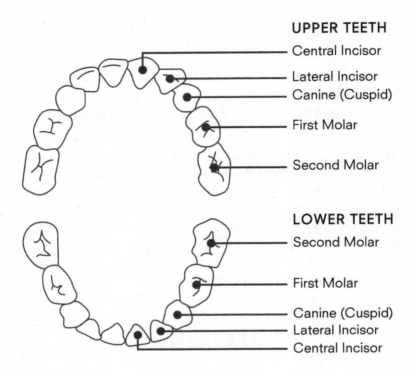

UPPER TEETH

Central Incisor

Lateral Incisor

Canine (Cuspid)

First Molar

Second Molar

LOWER TEETH

Second Molar

First Molar

Canine (Cuspid)

Lateral Incisor

Central Incisor

Most children will have all their milk teeth by the time they are between two and three years old.

You may have heard about the classic signs of teething, such as dribbling, putting anything and everything in their mouth, and chewing objects/toys. As teething is uncomfortable, babies do tend to be a little more unsettled or irritable. Their night-time sleep may also be disrupted and, during the day, they may need you to comfort them or distract them more. Teething can be tough on parents, too. Some say that nappy rash may be a sign of teething, but I'm not entirely convinced by this and think it's always best to explore other causes of nappy rash, such as diet or a bug, and introduce more nappy-free time and barrier cream.

'Home remedies often don't work, so we do say if your baby seems uncomfortable and in pain, then, as long as it is okay for them to have it, you may want to pick up paracetamol-based (baby-safe) medication to help. Paracetamol is a pain reliever. If the baby seems unwell, has a high temperature and you're worried about them, I would definitely recommend you get them checked.'

Laura Smith, specialist community public health nurse (health visitor) Ebonie Chandraraj, specialist community public health nurse (health visitor) @gentlehealthvisitors

Once teeth have come through, oral hygiene is important and you need to start cleaning your baby's tiny teeth. If they've only got a few teeth, silicone finger brushes are good or just a bit of cloth on your finger to wipe them over works too. Do be careful, though, as baby will likely bite down on your finger and this can be rather painful once they have a few teeth! Be very mindful of what you are putting in your baby's mouth and what they are consuming – adult toothpaste is not safe for babies. It contains too much fluoride so be sure to get an age-appropriate toothpaste that's as gentle as possible. You only need a very small smear of toothpaste at this stage. When they've got more teeth, you may want to graduate to a baby toothbrush – exciting times. These are often lovely and soft, and some are helpful shapes too as it can be hard to get around all the teeth. Babies at this age tend to swallow anything in their mouth and love to chew on a brush. Make sure you change the brush every few months and never leave them unattended with it. Dentists will recommend you brush their teeth twice a day, just like adults do.

THE ROLE OF YOUR HEALTH VISITOR

As your baby grows and develops, it is important to know that you still have healthcare professionals available to support the two of you. Lots of parents aren't aware that they can contact their health visitor from birth to age five. Health visitors can be a great resource and many have been midwives too. You can contact your health visitor by phone, and some teams now have mobile numbers, so you can send a text with your question, which can be easier when you have your hands full with a new baby!

Routine and finding your flow

MOTHERHOOD, MOST NOTABLY with the first child, is a fine balancing act between consciously striving to make things work in your adulting and going with the flow of their babying. In the first few months, it may feel as though you are surrendering to some level of chaos, due to the unpredictability of it all. Then many parents start to identify a pattern when their baby is around three to four months old. Sometimes this comes earlier, while for others it is later – again, there's no hard and fast rule, so try not to worry if you still haven't identified a pattern with your baby.

Two of the earliest patterns to spot are your baby's feeding and sleep–wake windows, which may start to rule your life around this time. This isn't always the case, though – some mums don't want to be confined to the home for their baby's naps and choose to encourage their baby to sleep in the pram or car; while others want to stick to a routine and have their baby nap in a dark room in their cot at home. You'll know what is right for your lifestyle and your family. No matter what anyone tells you, there is absolutely no right or wrong. Light routine may be helpful for predicting patterns for your baby, but some people want a set routine and others don't. You do what works for you and try not to worry too much about what everyone else is doing. It's easier said than done, I know, but once you've mastered the skill of caring less you'll feel a sense of lightness. One day you will feel like you're in the swing of things as you find *your* flow. And that's whatever's best for you and your baby.

HONESTY BOX

I did a bit of both. I would make an effort to get back home for nap times and stick to a routine. But we also travelled a lot to Cornwall (where I grew up), so we were on and off trains or in and out of the car and I couldn't always stick to our routine. That was my choice – I needed to see my family and prioritised my support network in Cornwall. While we were in Cornwall, I wanted to go for a nice beach walk or out for lunch with my family. I could easily get Georgie to sleep on me in the carrier or in the pram with some *shhh*ing and rocking – offering me the best of both worlds. Not all babies will be happy with this and for some the disruption in routine can cause distress.

Even as a routine starts to take shape, some days it will feel impossible to get out of the door and you might find yourself giving up on whatever you had planned. We've all been there several times – you aren't failing if this happens and it's okay to let the morning or afternoon slip away from you. Some days you have the energy to get up and out and leave plenty of time for the random events that occur during motherhood, and other times you just don't.

As a result of feeling under pressure, sometimes due to the wake window or lack of time to do anything at all, lots of mums find themselves rushing – sprinting upstairs to grab another muslin or that long-lost sock (how on earth do so many socks go missing? I counted 11 odd socks the other day). But there's really no need to put yourself under that level of pressure to get out of the home. Being flexible with your plans is key and so is looking after yourself in those moments of getting ready to go out. There is a lot to remember and consider – you're thinking for two or more people after all, depending on how many children you have and how supportive your partner is (no dig intended).

Often, rushing just makes you feel stressed.

Tip: One thing that does speed things up, if you have the energy for it, is planning the night before. This is something I am still learning the art of – organisation and thinking ahead! It's not a personal strength of mine, but it is a game-changer and makes mum life that little bit easier.

WHAT TO PACK WHEN LEAVING THE HOME

Something that can really help to ease the stress of going out is to always have a bag ready to go by the door. When you get back home, top it up with the bits you have used and leave it in a designated place for you and whoever is caring for your baby. I only started doing this around a year into motherhood but I *wish* I had got into the routine of this earlier.

Things to pack ready to go:

- Snacks and drinks for you – essential!
- Teething ring or age-appropriate toy/teddy that may help distract/comfort.
- A book – fabric books are best as they're lightweight and safer in the car.
- Muslin – to mop up the dribble, and any other bodily fluids often excreted by your baby (and sometimes you!).
- If bottle-feeding, the equipment you need.
- Wipes.
- Nappies – have five-plus in the bag and top up after a day out.
- Nappy bags – also for clothes covered in some form of bodily fluid/poo.
- Easy-wipe-down changing mat.
- Nappy cream (avoid double-dipping with the same finger to avoid spreading bacteria).
- Two changes of clothes for baby plus warm hat/gloves in winter.
- Sling – fabric slings are great at this age and are easy to transport.
- Baby paracetamol or ibuprofen (if you choose to give these to your baby).

This looks like a long list, but you won't need to top up most of it regularly once you have packed it all in the bag.

Tip: I once made the mistake of giving Georgie a paper book in the car. Within five minutes she was eating it and had a decent section of a page in her mouth. I had to quickly pull over in an awkward place to get it off her. Remember, whatever you give your baby at this age will likely end up in their mouth, so if you can't get to them easily it's best to avoid this when travelling.

TOYS AND ENTERTAINMENT

While we are on the topic of baby gear, the absolute truth is that babies do not need fancy toys or brand-new gadgets. In fact, one of the best ways to support your baby's development is free movement. Play gyms (the fancy term) or a mat with a few bits and bobs that are age-appropriate are perfect. A little later on – at around six months – objects in your kitchen cupboard, such as wooden spoons, plastic lids, pots and pans, will often do. At this age, your baby will love experimenting, seeing how they can create noises from objects and reactions from you. One of their all-time favourite games is to drop something on the floor and have you pick it up. They love it! These kinds of interactions are a baby's way of learning about the basic laws of the universe – like gravity, physics, material behaviour, and so much more. What may appear to be erratic and uncoordinated is in fact sophisticated play that aids brain development. It's a fascinating time for them and they're excited by the development of their new skills. It's magical to watch.

You'll likely notice that babies do not know or care whether or not they're wearing hand-me-downs or charity shop bargains; they have far too many other things to occupy them. The biggest need your baby has is to feel loved and secure. Alongside free movement, one of the best ways to help your baby develop motor and language skills is human connection and interaction. Simply by holding, singing, cuddling, responding and encouraging them, you are building on a secure attachment. Of course, it's great to have some toys for them to play with for those moments when you're not able to interact during the day, but try not to worry too much about what you have and haven't got. Nothing will ever replace your love.

Returning to exercise

I LOVE EXERCISING and work out frequently – it's so beneficial for us all and is an important part of long-term human health. Simply put, we need to move our bodies to keep well. The body really doesn't like being stagnant, and leading a sedentary lifestyle can cause significant problems. One of the main causes of back and neck pain isn't posture as you may think – it's often due to lack of mobility.

That said, exercise was the last thing on my mind after birth. As I go on to cover in the next chapter on sleep, I was simply surviving at one time and not thriving, which is why I've asked my friends, Clare Bourne, pelvic health physiotherapist, and Charlie Barker, founder of Bumps & Burpees, to provide you with some sound advice on returning to exercise. I'll give you the heads-up: none of it is daunting and it will help you to be kind to yourself.

Let's start with some top tips from Clare:

'Try to take the first six weeks after birth to rest, heal and recover, while taking care of your little one. This doesn't mean you can't be physically active in any way and start building some foundations for movement and exercise that you want to return to. Try starting with diaphragmatic breathing, pelvic floor exercises daily and short walks. Build your walks up slowly, and listen to any pain or discomfort you feel.

'After six weeks, you might feel really keen to get back to what you were doing before pregnancy or birth, but try to see the next six to eight weeks as an opportunity for really good rehabilitation and strengthening of the pelvic floor, abdominal muscles and other key muscles such as those in the bottom and legs. Start with body-weight movements such as squats and lunges, alongside low-impact exercise, for example cycling or swimming – postnatal Pilates or yoga are also recommended. Impact exercises like running or jumping, or lifting heavy weights, are usually advised to start gradually and slowly after around 12 weeks.

'There is no exact timescale we can all follow as we are all different. However, advice from the Department of Health recommends that new mums build up to 150 minutes of moderate-intensity activity a week, and encourages us that all activity counts.

'When returning to exercise, there are some symptoms to look out for and listen to. If you experience any incontinence, a heaviness sensation in the vagina, pain in the vagina, tummy or pelvis, or discomfort and/or pain in your C-section scar, this is feedback that the exercise you are doing might be a bit intense for your body right now. Sometimes we need to scale back slightly and take a bit longer to build up. It can feel frustrating, but don't push through symptoms. There is help for all these symptoms and seeing a pelvic health physiotherapist can help you to understand your body better.'

Clare Bourne, pelvic health physiotherapist

Charlie Barker adds:

'Don't rush. Whether you were super-fit before or even during your pregnancy, we can't forget that our body has been through something pretty extraordinary, so take your time and ease back into exercise steadily. When you are ready for some extra resistance, try adding in some light weights, whether that is with resistance bands or dumbbells, but again take it at a pace that feels comfortable for you and never be afraid to go back a step if it doesn't feel quite right.

'Don't compare. Whether you're comparing with someone else or your past self, it is not helpful for anyone because we are all on different journeys and we all recover at different rates, even from pregnancy to pregnancy, so listen to your body and do what feels good for you, not what someone else says should feel good.

'Let your past expectations go. Whether that is to do with the amount you exercise in a week, the things you achieve in that session, or even how you feel when you exercise. You are in a different phase of your life right now and things may be a bit different for a little while. We do not need to be adding guilt to our never-ending list of emotions, so if you can't fit in your workout today like you had planned because the day took a turn in a different direction, then simply draw a line under it and try again tomorrow.'

Charlie Barker, founder of Bumps & Burpees

Sleep

AS A SOCIETY our expectations of babies are often not in line with what is biologically normal. Some babies will sleep through the night very early on without the need for much support, but many won't – for some time, unless you support them to sleep with cuddles and rocking, co-sleep or sleep train them. There is a bit of stigma attached to older babies not sleeping through the night, or sometimes even mum-shaming. Your choices and views surrounding supporting your baby to sleep should be respected.

WHEN SHOULD A BABY SLEEP THROUGH THE NIGHT?

This is often the biggest question on exhausted new parents' minds. There are several considerations here. Let's start with the most common reason young babies wake during the night: to be fed. From *around* four to six months, excluding medical conditions or specific needs, *most* babies do not need to wake during the night for feeds. I suspect that is why some people expect a baby to sleep through from six months. Yet sleep is far more complex and, by focusing on their reduced feeding needs, we run the risk of overlooking other factors that impact infant sleep and cause disruptions – for example, routine, safety, the need to be comforted, temperament, sleep association, light, parents' stress levels, teething, life events, growth spurts, the fact they're a baby who's learning and so on. The simple fact is that some of us are better sleepers than others as adults and it's exactly the same for babies. They're all unique little people and all have their different needs. Sleep is not linear – it's ever-evolving and easily impacted, especially when babies are experiencing developmental leaps, are unwell or are teething. (We cover the most common illnesses on pages 190–95.)

The average amount of sleep a three-to-six-month-old baby needs is around 12–14 hours in a 24-hour period. This can vary significantly still, with some babies only wanting 10 hours and some 16. As with adults: we say the average person needs 6–8 hours, yet some live off 4 (I'm not sure how, but I know a few) and some (like my partner, Andy) prefer 10–11 hours.

In summary, like other topics we have discussed in the book, there is no hard and fast rule, no matter what the experts, other mums or society may tell you. Try to remove those expectations and look at your baby as an individual with unique needs. That way you can look at more appropriate ways to support them to sleep, rather than following a one-rule-fits-all approach.

THE DREAM FEED

A 'dream feed', where you gently rouse a baby but don't fully wake them for a feed just before you go to sleep, *may* encourage them to go longer in the night without waking for a feed. This can get that little bit more food in and enable a longer sleep for everyone. Nothing is ever guaranteed but it works a treat for some and is certainly worth considering.

'One of the most common concerns parents tend to have is surrounding sleep. Or lack of sleep. They think that, at three months old, their baby should be sleeping longer than two hours, but in lots of other cultures people realise that's not the norm. We try to empower parents to know that it's really normal for babies to wake up frequently way beyond three months.'

Laura Smith, specialist community public health nurse (health visitor) Ebonie Chandraraj, specialist community public health nurse (health visitor) @gentlehealthvisitors

UNDERSTANDING YOUR BABY'S SLEEP PATTERN

The term 'circadian rhythm' is used in reference to the natural workings of our body and the response we have to day and night. The word 'circadian' comes from Latin, *circa*, meaning 'around', and *dies*, meaning 'day'. It's a natural internal cycle that helps us wake up in the morning and sleep at night. As you may already know, throughout the day melatonin levels increase (a hormone your body produces to support and help induce sleep). Melatonin levels are impacted by light, which is one of the reasons many experts recommend getting as much daylight as possible and ensuring the room or environment is dark when you put your baby down to sleep. This is a signal to the body and supports it to know when to remain alert and when to sleep. Working with your natural circadian rhythm is a key milestone because sleep affects every aspect of your life.

Your baby's sleep–wake cycle starts to develop naturally from *around* eight weeks, though you won't be able to see any signs of it as it is more of an internal process. Your encouragement to slowly build a light framework of a sleep routine will likely help, and you can start working on eventually firming up a more robust routine as your baby grows and you get into your own flow.

Firstly, your baby needs to start to learn the difference between night and day. By making a point of 'bedtime', you can mark it with some signs and signals for your baby to begin to pick up on. They will learn that, at night, things become calmer and quieter, with less light. By lowering the lighting and sitting quietly giving your baby their evening feed, they will come to recognise the cues – becoming part of their bedtime routine. Some parents like to bath their baby before bed. I personally found baths stimulating for Georgie and avoided daily bathing as it can dry the skin out; your baby may well be different, though. Whatever you decide to include as part of your bedtime routine, keep it consistent, relaxed and gentle.

BABY BATH TIME

You may have decided not to over-wash your baby, giving their skin a chance to remain as natural as possible, for as long as possible. By 12 weeks most parents have decided it's time for a bath, but not all do want to – there is no pressure to get the bubble bath out. If you're keeping your baby clean with a top-to-toe, that's usually enough. If you do choose to bathe, you and your baby can share bath time together, assuming you have a bath, which can take the pressure off having to securely hold your baby while leaning over the bath. Be very mindful of the ingredients in any soaps or bubble baths – try to opt for natural soaps with minimal ingredients and without harsh chemicals. Young babies don't really get dirty and by soaping them often you can dry out the skin and expose them to chemicals unnecessarily. Some babies love water and will really want to splash around, while others may take a while to enjoy bath time.

Always make sure you put the cold water in first and add hot water afterwards – you can use your elbow to check the temperature of the water or pick up a special bath thermometer that will alert you if the water is too hot. As you put the hot water in last, remember some may dribble out so keep your baby clear of the taps or run a little cold through to prevent hot water coming into contact with your baby's skin. You may also want to get your baby used to having a splash and getting a bit of water near their head and face using your hand as a cup. They may need reassurance and calming strokes while you do this, or they may be totally okay with it. They're all so different! If not already, gradually they will start to feel more relaxed and confident in water.

SLEEP TRAINING

Between three and six months may seem quite early on to be talking about sleep training, but I think it's important to mention it here as some people do want to start implementing some baby-led methods to begin laying the foundations of sleep support around this time, while others opt for controlled crying. Whether you decide to sleep train (which usually involves putting your baby down in a safe place to sleep without your assistance via rocking, holding, feeding, and so on) or not is a very individual choice.

Experts say different things about sleep training and, once again, there is a wide spectrum of views. As parents you need to find where you sit on that spectrum. Some people adopt fairly firm viewpoints, such as 'Never let a baby cry', while for others, 'Protest crying is fine,' and a smaller group says, 'Leave them to cry it out entirely, they learn quickest that way.' What you decide is right for you and your baby very much depends on temperament – yours and your baby's – your lifestyle, situation, personal experiences, beliefs, culture, previous experiences with babies, work commitments and mental health, to name a few.

HONESTY BOX

I've got a confession: before I had Georgie, I assumed any form of sleep training was the last thing I'd do. I could not comprehend how or why anyone would let their baby cry in any capacity. Then I had a baby and still thought that for around seven months. By then, I had been kept awake pretty much every single night – sometimes for minutes, sometimes for hours, for months on end. I was utterly exhausted and couldn't remember who I was anymore. Although it wasn't that many months before, my life pre-baby was a distant memory. I was a totally different person; someone I could not relate to at all. Now everything was hazy, making decisions was more difficult than ever, I was very irritable, tearful, and needed a lot of sugar and caffeine to get through the day. I gained weight and felt sluggish. Even on the days when I was a shell of a person, if I lounged on the sofa for longer than an hour I felt guilty for not getting up and out because Georgie had big, big energy and I was obsessed with her getting 'fresh air'. Exhaustion became the new normal and the most accurate description of night-time for me during the first seven months is: traumatic. I completely changed my view and could now see why parents would opt to sleep train. At the time I wondered if this was my life forever now, if either she or I would ever sleep through the night again. If you're there, I am so sorry you're experiencing this difficulty. Sleep deprivation is a form of torture. I promise it will end. They do eventually sleep – whatever you choose to do. *You will sleep through the night again.*

When it comes to sleep training, it's best to avoid becoming fixated on one ideology – like I did. Convincing yourself that one specific way is the only way can cause you a lot of distress, especially if you change your mind. Give yourself permission to adapt and be compassionate towards yourself if you move in another direction. We all have ideas about what we will be like as mothers and sometimes, when faced with a situation, we behave in a different way. Please try not to judge yourself if that happens – honestly, we all do it! All babies are different and your experience with this baby will be different to that of your friend, cousin, neighbour, or the influencer sharing her story online.

SLEEP CONSULTANTS

There are many sleep consultants out there, some providing face-to-face support, others online, and some with on-demand courses. Like many parents do, if you choose to seek professional support from a sleep consultant, ensure they are appropriately qualified and ideally have decent experience. Below are a few red flags to look out for:

- Suggesting that you wean early to improve sleep.
- Guaranteeing results.
- Recommending anything that goes against The Lullaby Trust's advice (see pages 100–103).
- Suggesting anything that's judgemental and based on personal opinion rather than fact – watch out for this one!
- If your gut tells you not to follow their advice.

COMPARISON IS THE THIEF OF JOY

If you were to compare your baby to your friends' or family's babies (or anyone else's for that matter), you'd soon start to worry about something. There will always be differences because they are different people.

Comparison is part of human nature and enables us to feel part of a group or social network. It's a very natural thing for us to do as mothers – we sometimes want validation and we often want confirmation that everything is well. Comparison can be a way of assessing whether or not you're doing the 'right' thing and your baby is 'normal'. Being inquisitive, inspired or asking for tips is different to comparing. In motherhood it's always best to ensure you remain inquisitive rather than worrying about the differences between babies.

I know this, but I still couldn't help comparing Georgie's sleep needs.

HONESTY BOX

Georgie wouldn't nap during the day for longer than 30–45 minutes and had a lot of energy. She would start her day around 5.30am and be non-stop. I couldn't take my eyes off her. She sat up unattended at 16 weeks, skipped crawling entirely, was cruising by six months (where babies hold on to a table or the sofa to cruise around) and walking by ten months. I was so very happy for her that she did things early, but it felt like I was in a time machine and her needs changed so fast by the day – I couldn't keep up. I was feeling really fed up with Georgie's low sleep needs and the lack of time I had to do anything. I'd ask friends for help, in a desperate attempt to fix Georgie's sleep, 'So, please tell me exactly what you do,' and they'd say, 'No different to what you do; they're just good sleepers, Marie.'

And that was the truth of the matter. It took me a while, but I eventually learnt to accept that I had a baby with low sleep needs and I would get more rest again one day. I learnt to ask for more help and delegate tasks. I also learnt to be more realistic with my time-planning – 30 minutes goes very quickly, so first thing in the morning I wrote a little list of the essentials required within that half-hour. Or, even better, I allowed myself to rest.

As with feeding, sometimes parents feel pressured to pick a side – usually either sleep training or co-sleeping (see pages 103–4). You do not have to do this. You can adapt to suit your lifestyle and, most importantly, you can do what you think is right for your family at the time, trusting your instincts. People can become very pushy with their opinions and perception of what is right for other families. While this is often done with good intentions and usually with the belief they're helping, you are particularly vulnerable and can be misled by someone else's ideas when framed in a certain way.

The bottom line is: **your family set-up and needs will lead you to make a decision about sleeping arrangements and supporting your baby to sleep that best suits you**. Try not to feel embarrassed about what you have chosen to do – you're not doing anything 'wrong'. Only you know what feels right and is best.

Relationship difficulties

LOTS OF MUMS tell me they weren't prepared for the detrimental effect having a baby would have on their relationship, so I want to talk about that for a moment and address how you might be feeling. Ultimately, you're not alone if you have become unhappy in your relationship – it's extremely common. The stats opposite are based on heterosexual partnerships. At this time, we don't have much research on same-sex partnerships. One study included 218 couples spanning the first eight years of marriage and concluded that parenthood significantly impacts marital function. These changes were reported to be sudden and to persist over time.

It is so very important that we delve into these sudden changes. I do not have all the answers for your relationship, but I do have some healthy suggestions that have been studied and appear to work. If you're struggling at the moment, I know how hard it really is for you. You may feel anything from slightly dissatisfied to fantasising about leaving your partner, or worse!

'I literally wanted to punch my husband in the face on a daily basis. If I didn't have the baby in my arms I think I would have done, on a few occasions. He was so selfish and I had to state the obvious all the time, usually starting with "Can you help me/pass me . . ." I felt really alone during our struggles and lost confidence in us as a couple. We were so in love, why did no one tell me about the divide having a baby would create between us? It was a huge shock and I thought it was just us struggling. I hated him for almost a year, until we had counselling. It wasn't easy to get back, but I do love him dearly again. We needed support to understand each other's needs as parents rather than husband and wife. We are having another baby and things will be ever so different this time.'

Anonymous, mum of one, expecting baby number two

THE OVERLOAD FOR MODERN MUMS

Modern mums have an increasing variety of equal opportunities and choice of roles on offer in the workplace – including leadership positions. It's fantastic to see. In comparison, our foremothers had to deal with inequality to the extent of having to accept situations such as legalised rape and other forms of abuse – simply because they were married. Some parts of the world did, and still do, normalise and accept inequality and injustices in relationships. Thankfully, attitudes are, overall, changing for the better.

It's a bittersweet time as the parameters of 'roles at home' have become blurred, but the modern mum often juggles a lot. The list is long and often includes things like event organiser, admin support, family diary manager, family liaison coordinator, playmate, entertainer, counsellor, shopper, cleaner, night watcher and sometimes breadwinner too. This means we need to be mindful of how we expend our energy. If we're not careful and attempt to continue to do it all, we can and likely will burn out or become depleted at some point. At the least, we can find ourselves run ragged, unwell or exhausted – a different version of ourselves. When employment is thrown into the mix, the balance is generally still tipped in favour of men. Not only do I hear this anecdotally on a regular basis, but it's reflected in data from the Office for National Statistics:

- In April to June 2021, 3 in 4 mothers with dependent children were in work in the UK, reaching its highest level in the equivalent quarter over the last 20 years.
- In March 2022, employed women with dependent children spent more time on unpaid childcare (an average of 85 minutes per day) and household work (an average of 167 minutes per day) than employed men with dependent children (56 and 102 minutes per day, respectively).
- From 2020, in families where both parents are employed, it has become more common for both parents to work full-time, rather than a man working full-time with a partner working part-time.

HONESTY BOX

I couldn't help but notice some of the disparities and unfair balance in my own experiences of motherhood. Things were off balance and I became terribly unhappy, angry and frustrated with Andy. I was doing way too much and spreading myself far too thin. Many mums have no choice but to work. I didn't have a choice either and had to go back to work while breastfeeding, which we delve into on pages 223–5. There came a point for me when I had a 'make or break' crisis – something had to be done.

Depending on your support network, the workload varies from person to person. It's important to build relationships with your tribe in general, but especially with your support person at home, so that there's a fair and equal balance. When I say equal I don't mean a 50/50 split on childcare specifically. It's more about equally supporting the family – whatever that may look like for you. Some mums want to spend way more than 50 per cent of their share with their baby and need relief from other tasks in order to do this. Others want a fairer split around childcare.

TAKING OWNERSHIP

Taking ownership of new responsibilities may not be something that comes naturally to some partners. It's not just them being lazy (maybe for some it is – I'll recuse myself here and let you be the judge of that); perhaps they genuinely do not know what you need support with and where they now fit in. New babies bring about new people after all, and it takes time for you all to settle in. You often have different priorities and more decisions to make, as a couple. Naturally, one of you takes the lead on this and that is usually you, mama, especially in the first year.

HONESTY BOX

Since having Georgie, I have fallen out of love and back in love with Andy. I felt very distant from him at times and my expectations did not meet my reality. That's not to say he did anything wrong – he didn't. Nonetheless, the expectation versus reality can be a hard pill to swallow and can make you feel lonely sometimes – even when you're in the same room. We argued a lot during that first year. I expected him to know what I needed, and learnt that he needed me to say exactly what I needed, rather than shouting it three days later during an argument.

Research shows that the majority of parents argue more during the first year than at any other time, so we weren't unusual. I expected Andy to do certain things and he assumed I was happily doing those same things. In reality, I was becoming more and more exhausted and unhappy, until resentment took over my feelings towards him. I will admit it got so bad that I struggled to see him having fun because I could barely pee in peace, let alone take part in leisure activities – what the hell was leisure anymore? He would 'pop off' to play golf for a few hours, while I ploughed my way through a very long to-do list as well as breastfed and entertained Georgie. I missed several dental appointments; accidentally used dishwasher tablets in the washing machine a few times while in a sleep-deprived haze; often forgot to book Georgie's music class and turned up anyway, hoping they would let me in; needed to go shopping (always); realised Georgie's babygrows were getting a bit tight, and forgot my own mum's birthday. That's just to give a few examples.

At times, I viciously lashed out because I felt jealous of Andy's freedom. It was hard to accept that my life had changed in every way possible. Yet his life appeared hardly to change at all. He slept through the night while I breastfed, he drank beer while I drove, wore nice clothes while I wore unflattering feeding-friendly tops decorated with leaked milk patches or one of Georgie's bodily fluids. It seemed so unfair and I felt defeated, fed up with my new yet permanent and relentless 'mum duty'. As new parents, it seemed like we had very different perspectives on life.

This is all deeply personal and I have chosen to be completely honest with you about how I felt and how I initially managed those feelings, which was unhealthy. And I am admitting that to you because I'd rather share my mistakes and help us learn from them together.

As a culture I don't think we are open enough about the challenges couples face after having children. I have spoken to many, many mums who have been with their partners for many years, virtually argument-free. Yet, after having a baby, suddenly arguing becomes the new norm. Everywhere we look, we see a lot of 'happy' couples posting shots of their rosy family life or date nights – all smiles for the camera. There's nothing wrong with sharing these images, but when you're going through a rough patch with your other half, seeing 'perfection' in other couples can make you feel more alone in the difficulties you're facing in your own relationship. When I have been open and honest on- and offline, I've had so many responses that have confirmed without doubt why we must talk about these challenges more.

If you find yourself nodding your head in recognition and relating to the above, one of the biggest dilemmas is what to do about the situation. Everyone is different and relationships are complex because the human brain, interactions and emotions are all very complex in their own right. What works for me may not work for you. In fact, you might not have any axes to grind and may be one of the lucky mums who cannot relate to any of the difficulties I faced. But for those who are interested in addressing these issues, I'd like to offer a solution that worked for Andy and me, backed by research.

DEFINING ROLES AND RESPONSIBILITIES

Like a new job in the workplace, we (I) set out roles and responsibilities based on the new demands we had as parents. Then we took on tasks that we were both happy with and wrote them down. I still have the A4 sheet of paper in my bedside cabinet with our names assigned to responsibilities. I even asked Andy to sign it, and I did too.

That may seem a bit over the top and too formal for some, but I wanted to make everything crystal clear. If you can see it explicitly written down, it doesn't sound like nagging if you ask them to fulfil what they've signed up to. We agreed to share even the simplest tasks and that meant a lot to me. For example, Andy now cooks and does bedtime two evenings a week, and I do the remainder. I do the food shopping and he does the car/household maintenance, like taking out the bins/meter readings, etc. I hate vacuuming and he is happy to do it. We learnt how to work as a team, which took some of the load from me. This allowed me some breathing space and made me feel supported. It was one of the best things I instigated for myself as a mum – defined and delegated support.

The concept of treating parenthood like a job with set roles and responsibilities may not work for everyone, but it might be worth a try and could help you get the solid support you deserve. If both partners are working, both need to get decent rest – somehow. Sleep, rest and relaxation are vital for a healthy mind and relationship. There is so much focus on the baby and you give so much of yourself as a mother to this little person you've brought into the world. Sometimes it's hard to give any more to anyone else and it's easy to forget each other. Yet by creating some space for yourself, you're better able to respond to your partner and keep the fire going. Relationships need maintenance – pre-baby you may not have noticed this as much, or it may have come more naturally.

As life with a baby is ever-evolving, there may be times when you feel the workload is becoming unbalanced, or perhaps you'll have another baby and it'll be time to have another look at the task allocation. It's worth the extra attention and the time it takes to bring any imbalances to the forefront and have a rethink. Try to avoid letting things go, as, more often than not, you don't really let them go. Instead, you'll likely let resentment build and you need to make sure you feel things are fair in your relationship. You are so worthy of that, mama – speak up and be open about what you need.

Tired or resentful parents can become unreasonable, like I did, and I regret a lot of my behaviour around that time in my life. I regret what I did not say more than I regret the things I did – and I said some harsh things. As a couple, it's important to tell each other how well you're both doing and to reconnect too. Time out is what all parents need – from a 20-minute coffee to date nights or even a mini break . . . whatever you're able to fit in. Factoring in time together will go a long way to helping you get back on track and falling in love with the new person you're now with: the parent version of your partner.

IF IT'S STILL NOT WORKING

As important as working on your relationship may be, sadly some couples just cannot find a way through. This can be heartbreaking, but I don't want to avoid talking about it. Sometimes ending the relationship is for the best. The only ones who know whether or not they can make it work, or want to make it work, are you and your partner. People may offer advice or push you towards what they think is best, but they may not really understand. You deserve to be happy, and to feel appreciated and comfortable with the person you have chosen to spend your life with.

In some very sad cases, leaving a partner may be the safest option for you and your baby. Abuse comes in many forms within relationships and 'domestic violence' has since been amended to the more accurate description 'domestic abuse'. Not all abuse is physical; much of it can be emotional, psychological or financial and, mama, you do not need to live with it. I know, it's unbelievably tough when someone has squashed your self-worth or made you believe you need them because no one else will want you. Or made you think you could not live without them. None of it is true. None of it. More often than not, this type of coercive control is based on the perpetrator's fear of you rebuilding your confidence, seeing them for what they are – then leaving them. If you're experiencing any form of abuse, it's not your fault, you will not be judged, and there are many safe places and charities where you can seek help, such as Refuge, Women's Aid or the National Domestic Abuse Helpline (see pages 242–3). Pick up the phone and call – you and your baby both deserve better and to be safe from harm.

SOLO PARENTING

~~~

However you come to solo parenting, whether it's from day one and opting for a sperm donor or going your separate ways after splitting with your partner further down the line, it can be a tough yet incredible journey. I've met ever so many mums who are solo parenting and they have all said very similar things – relaying the importance of their social network and support. Finding a 'tribe' for all mums is important, but even more so for those who are single. This is because you need to be able to speak to someone about how you feel, to vent and share experiences; you need someone to walk through this journey with. Other mums experiencing similar situations can lift you up when you're feeling low and provide comfort like no one else can. The power of true empathy here goes a very long way.

Female ties and friendships are incredible and mums often build bonds with each other very quickly. One mum once told me she replaced her partner with another single mum and they ended up parenting both their young children together. They would have childcare swaps so they could go on nights out, text each other pictures of their kids doing funny things throughout the day (like they would a partner), and share a good old rant about their troubles. She explained to me that what was initially a very scary time ended up becoming a relief: free from her unpleasant partner, she was then able to build a beautiful friendship she would never have had the opportunity to pursue had she not become single.

Gingerbread, a fantastic charity for single parents, has a wealth of information on their website and a helpline (see page 245). They also offer the option to become a member, introducing you to thousands of other single parents.

KEY POINTS

- Some days will pass you by. Try not to rush and put additional pressure on yourself.
- Being organised in advance really does help, when you have the energy for it.
- Sleep is complex. Your decision regarding sleeping arrangements or sleep support may change. It's okay to adapt to your needs as mum life unfolds.
- There's a huge developmental leap between three and six months. Some experts claim it is one of the biggest and most difficult, so hang on in there. This too shall pass.
- Relationship difficulties affect the majority of couples after having a baby. Assigning roles and responsibilities fairly may help.
- Communication and shared responsibility for tasks within the home may lead to a healthier, more manageable balance for you. Speak up rather than expect help.

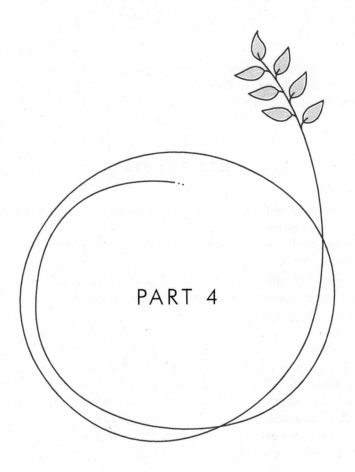

PART 4

Six to Nine Months

~~~~~~

The six-to-nine-month period sees better communication between you and your baby, bringing your worlds a little closer. Your baby will now be able to experience the joy of food. By nine months, your baby might be pointing and giving you further clues to their preferences. It's a beautiful time as you watch your baby progress.

In this section, once we've looked at what to expect from this age, we will start off with what I'm sure is at the forefront of your mind – weaning! We'll then move on to other milestones, such as cruising and crawling, travelling with your baby and, finally, the most common childhood illnesses in the under-ones.

What to expect

AS MENTIONED PREVIOUSLY, it is important to follow your baby's inner timeline – they all do different things at different times, and that's okay. Below are some ideas of behaviours and physical developments you might see emerging from six months onwards, though this is by no means set in stone:

- Sitting up without support.
- Recognising words or their name.
- Babbling, gurgling, making sounds and copying sounds more accurately.
- Pulling themselves up to cruise.
- Showing signs of teething: dribbling, biting and appearing to be in discomfort.
- 'Cutting' their first tooth.
- If you sign, they may recognise more signs or start to sign back.
- Showing interest in food.
- By nine months, they may be crawling, cruising and even walking!

SPATIAL AWARENESS

During this time, your baby becomes more aware of the distance between themselves and people and objects. They will start to work out that you are able to walk away and leave them. Even if they are on the move and crawling, they won't yet be able to catch up with you. This can be a little scary for them and you may notice your baby keeping an eye on you, checking to see where you are. Watching you and checking your whereabouts may start before six months and last way past nine months of age. It's very common and normal behaviour.

SPEECH AND BABBLING

~~~

Although your baby is not quite ready to progress into the world of verbal communication, they are learning and preparing for it. You may notice more babbling or different noises coming from your baby. They are exploring the various ways they can create sound through their vocal systems. Appearing impressed with their sounds will support and encourage them to continue this exploration. Yet again, you really don't need to do anything major – they're learning from you and your conversations all the time.

Rhythmicity of communication between you two builds on their conversational skills. By this, I mean taking turns in a rhythm: they babble, pause, you respond, pause and so on. By nine months they may be able to associate words with meaning, the most common being 'bye-bye' accompanied by waving.

CONNECTION BETWEEN YOU AND YOUR BABY

~~~

You and your baby don't exist as isolated beings because each of you is impacted by the other. Although your baby has been outside of your body for some time, they are still very reliant on you for so much, especially learning about communication. Equally, you are impacted by your baby's communication with you, which is one of the reasons motherhood can be so intense. Often your bodies will sync, so your heart-rate patterns of acceleration and deceleration will mimic each other, without you even realising it.

Even though visually you appear to be separate, your body and brains are still very closely interlinked and you have learnt specific communications – from noises to facial expressions – that no one else may be able to pick up on. There are many layers of communication you and your baby will continue to build on while your baby is developing their social brain and beginning to understand relationships.

Tip: Where possible, get someone to take little videos of you together or take some yourself – these are such precious memories to look back on. One popped up on my phone recently and it made me cry; just me and Georgie poking out our tongues at each other, but you can see the light of connection in our eyes and it's magical to be able to watch this almost as an outsider at a later date. You can forget about these moments in and among the chaos.

OTHER BEHAVIOURAL CHANGES

As your baby is starting to understand more about how the world works, they may be a little more wilful or expressive. Changing their nappy may become a battle as they realise they can kick and wriggle away. This can be frustrating for you – especially when poo is being smeared across their toe or your hand (been there!). Distractions are a great tactic to help you get on and change them. Babies may also thrash around more in their sleep and have some difficulty getting off to sleep as they turn their head from side to side. This is usually normal behaviour as they try to get comfortable. Lastly, an attachment to a particular toy or teddy may start to form, or just wanting to hold something as they go about their day for comfort. Georgie always had to have something in her hand.

BUILDING ON MOTOR SKILLS

At around this age, babies are far better coordinated and may be able to copy some of your body movements too. They begin to master the pincer grasp (see pages 178–9) and explore new ways of moving their body. Their hands are tools that empower them to discover the world and they go from staring at toys or others playing to wanting to get involved themselves. Most babies want to get their hands on anything and everything in sight. One of the best ways to encourage this is free movement and free play in a safe place with age-appropriate toys. Messy play can be great for this. We had a local group we went to, which saved me having to clean up after at home.

THE NEED TO NAP

Sleeping is important because doubling your brain size within a year is energy-consuming stuff. Sleeping is a way of processing information and there's an awful lot of information to process. To put things into context, an adult brain uses up around 20 per cent of energy input, whereas a baby's uses up to 65 per cent. Some experts report even more than this. The rapid growth and vast amount to learn is exhausting – leading them to nap. One study found that having an extended nap of 30 minutes or more within 4 hours of learning a set of object–action pairings from a puppet toy enabled 6- and 12-month-old infants to retain their memories of new behaviour. These findings support the view that the frequency of napping may play an essential role in babies establishing long-term memory.

The average sleep need at this stage is similar to 3–6 months, at around 12–14 hours in a 24-hour period. Remember, we are all different and this is a rough guide. Some babies have high sleep needs; others have lower.

While we are on the subject of sleep, as mentioned on page 101 it's safest to have your baby sleep in the same room as you until the age of 6 months. Thereafter, you may (or may not) want to put your baby in a separate bedroom in a cot. Do what feels right for you and your family in terms of sleeping arrangements. Please don't feel pressured or rushed into getting them out of your room if it doesn't feel right. Trust your own instincts here and be sure to follow The Lullaby Trust's safer sleep advice (see pages 100–103). You may also want to get a baby monitor so you can still see your baby when they do sleep in a separate room. There are many on the market – we bought the cheapest one that enabled me to see and hear Georgie.

SEPARATION ANXIETY

~~~~

Between the ages of six and 12 months, the social part of the brain develops significantly in volume and connectivity. This is a universal finding for babies in all cultures globally. Prior to their ability to use language to communicate or confirm their thoughts, they need to rely on an attachment to their main caregivers. Around this time babies may experience separation anxiety as they want to be around the people they know meet their needs and keep them safe. As a result, a seemingly outgoing baby may become clingy or easily upset. This can worry parents or lead them to question whether something else is wrong, like teething for example. This is always a possibility, but it's also very likely their social brain is making sense of relationships and they crave the safety of their mum.

Weaning

AS WITH SO many other baby-related things, parents have different approaches, attitudes and feelings towards weaning. Some are excited and eager, others are anxious, and some are sad that their baby is growing up fast and that this stage has come around so quickly. If you have been breastfeeding, you might find this change liberating. Equally, it can feel like added pressure for some mums. Gone are the days when your boob covered breakfast, lunch and dinner.

Note for breastfeeding mamas: As your baby starts to eat solid food regularly, you will likely notice a change in the supply of your breast milk. As time goes on, your body will adjust, reducing milk production as the need for it declines. This is all a healthy and normal process – you don't need to worry about it as your body will adjust naturally with your baby's needs.

Food is more than nutrition to many of us; it brings us pleasure and sensory stimulation as we see, smell, taste and explore textures. The smells of food pass through the olfactory bulb in the brain and are linked to memories and emotions, and certain foods can take us back to a place or people – like our grandparents' signature dish or a meal we had on holiday, for example. Eating is often a way of marking social occasions or celebrations. This human behaviour – or ritual, as many may say – is observed globally. Most nations mark celebrations with or have ceremonies around food and have done for centuries.

Mealtimes give us the opportunity to spend (ideally) uninterrupted quality time together. As your baby enters the realm of eating, they too can enjoy these experiences, depending on your cultural background or social norms. In my home, during mealtimes, we try not to have phones at the dinner table, and we try as much as possible to take time, relax and enjoy our meals as well as each other's company. It's not always like this. We certainly aren't the perfect family and sometimes I do allow Georgie to sit with the TV on and eat while I get on with something urgent or finish work. But we try to make that the exception.

Not everyone finds mealtimes easy. Sadly, some parents have had or still have a difficult relationship with food. The UK charity Beat (formerly Eating Disorders Association) estimates that around 1.25 million people in the UK have an eating disorder – with 75 per cent of those affected being female. Parents who are affected by eating disorders could find that this time triggers previous issues or exacerbates current disorders. If this is the case, you may want to address any issues by seeking advice from Beat (see page 243) or your GP so that you can have a more enjoyable time around food and weaning your baby.

SETTING UP

Being prepared with equipment and knowledge is one way to support you to feel calm about this stage, so let's start with the basics. You'll need:

- Some bibs (which might include a wipeable plastic one that catches the food).
- Baby-safe cutlery – there are now some brilliant designs and eco-friendly items on the market, or the bog-standard cheap and cheerful ones, depending on your budget.
- A highchair – there are different designs here: some are standalone with their own little table and others just have a chair that you position at your family dining table. We bought a second-hand one which had barely been used and was less than half the original price. Used equipment isn't for everyone and you may prefer a new chair. Either way, your baby should be able to sit independently with control over their head and neck when in the chosen chair. (Note: babies should never be left unattended in the highchair.)

Weaning is an exciting time indeed for babies, full of exploration and curiosity. They will often play with food, dropping it on themselves, on the floor, or throwing it around. Watching your walls getting splattered with food you've spent time and effort to prepare or buy is less exciting for you. We got a huge dollop of spinach mixed with breast milk over our cream sofa within the first week of weaning (and quickly changed where we positioned the highchair!).

VITAMINS

The government recommends that all children aged six months to five years are given daily vitamin supplements that come in oral drop form and contain vitamins A, C and D. Babies who are having more than 500ml (about a pint) of infant formula a day should not be given vitamin supplements. This is because formula is fortified with vitamins A, C and D and other nutrients.

THE BIGGEST FEAR

Many parents say that they are fearful of their baby choking during the weaning stage. I was no exception. It's not a nice thought and a very normal fear, but I want to reassure you that choking is rare when you follow the safety tips around food. Knowing exactly what to do can really help alleviate some of the anxiety when it comes to weaning.

There's a big difference between choking and gagging, but they're often confused. Gagging is an inbuilt defence mechanism to help prevent choking. Babies have a particularly sensitive gag reflex that can be triggered closer to the front of the tongue than in adults. Babies haven't yet developed the ability to properly coordinate chewing. It takes around four years for us to master the ability to manoeuvre food to the back of our mouth to swallow. The gag reflex kicks in when needed and is a cleverly designed neuro-muscular safety measure.

It can be difficult not to be fearful when your baby gags during the weeks of weaning, but this is very common and usually normal. When gagging, your baby will retch for a moment and go on to breathe as normal, maintaining good oxygen levels and therefore a healthy skin colour. Babies are usually unfazed by gagging and will happily continue to eat. As your baby grows, they will gag less and the reflex will move more towards the back of the mouth. If you are ever worried about your baby's gag reflex, give your GP a call, as some have an oversensitive reflex and your GP may offer to refer you to a specialist if necessary.

Choking is different to gagging and often needs your immediate intervention. When choking, babies cough and they may be able to successfully expel the food (or object) themselves. If they are **unable to cough, speak or cry** or appear blue around the lips, you will need to intervene. There are also things you can do to prevent choking (see a list of foods you should avoid offering whole on page 181). Guidelines also advise that babies aren't to be left alone while eating. Of course, accidents can still happen, so for safety I highly recommend every new parent attend a first-aid course. There are several available, from online to in-person, and lots of free resources on the Resuscitation Council website too (see page 243).

THE ANATOMY BIT

The mouth, jaw, throat and oesophagus are all part of a truly fascinating collaboration of bodily functions. There are around 50 muscles available to be called upon just to get a mouthful of food from your mouth to your stomach. The mechanics required to support swallowing ensure the input (hopefully something delicious) is distributed to the correct place. Take a breath in now, hold it, swallow, and then breathe out. This seemingly simple and effortless process involves your throat directing and redirecting air as well as saliva through the epiglottis. The epiglottis is a small structure that is usually upright at rest, which allows air to pass into the larynx and lungs. When we swallow, it folds backwards to cover the entrance to the larynx, so that food and liquids don't enter the trachea (windpipe) and lungs. After swallowing, the epiglottis returns to its upright position. The human body and the daily tasks it performs for us with no additional instruction are often taken for granted (guilty). But the effortlessness of these tasks for us on a conscious level hides a great deal of complexity. The human body really is extraordinary.

WHEN IS THE BEST TIME TO START WEANING?

All babies are different and some are ready slightly sooner than others. The NHS, the Department of Health and the WHO recommend weaning a baby at around six months. Yet research by the Office for Health Improvement and Disparities (OHID) found that 40 per cent of first-time mums introduce solid food by the time their baby is five months old and almost two-thirds (64 per cent) say they have received conflicting advice on the best age to start weaning.

'I was shocked when they said the baby's not weaning – I thought, "She's almost five months old! What are you feeding her?" Apparently that's all changed now. Nothing like what I did with mine. I had six kids in eight years. We gave them all baby rice at around four months. I think my youngest might have had it at about three months. But she was a terrible sleeper and I was told to give her the baby rice to settle her down at night.'

Anonymous, grandma of three

Weaning a baby to support sleep may be advised by well-meaning family and friends, or even professionals, but most experts advise avoiding weaning until the baby is physically ready for food (see below).

SIGNS YOUR BABY IS READY

- Around six months of age.
- Sitting up unattended, with good control over head and neck.
- Able to bring an object to their mouth without your guidance.
- Reduction in tongue thrusting. If you touch their bottom lip with your finger or a spoon, do they stick their tongue out or open their mouth? Tongue thrusting is a sign they're not yet ready to swallow and more likely to push food out of the mouth.

Watching and being intrigued by your eating is normal for babies, but they need to be ready to wean. It's best to look at the visible physical signs and reflexes. These are slightly more reliable indicators than behaviour alone. If I had focused on behavioural signs exclusively, I would have weaned Georgie at around three months. She would stare at us as we ate from a very young age and try to grab food by four months. But physically I knew her body was not ready for food and waited until she displayed all the signs, which, in her case, was at around five and a half months.

You might be wondering what to do if your baby is displaying signs they're ready to wean at less than six months. Parents may mistake the behaviours listed below as indicators that their baby is ready for solid foods:

- chewing their fists
- waking up in the night (more than usual)
- wanting extra milk feeds

Most experts agree that it is not safe to wean earlier than 17 weeks. The OHID states: 'The introduction of solid foods may reduce the amount of breast milk consumed and is associated with greater risks of infectious illness in infants. Giving solid foods to breastfed infants before six months may also reduce breast milk intake without increasing total energy intake or increasing weight gain.'

Milk should remain a substantial part of a baby's diet until the age of one. Snacks between 'meals' are therefore not recommended until your baby is over one. Instead, milk should be offered. Both breast and formula milk contain loads of vitamins and nutrients to support your baby's development. Breast milk also contains lots of immune-boosting properties that help to protect your baby from illness. For this reason, some refer to weaning as 'complementary feeding'. Early on, the introduction of food should be *alongside* milk rather than a replacement for it.

THE 'PALMER GRASP' VERSUS THE 'PINCER GRASP'

At six months, your baby will be using the palmer grasp. This is when several fingers curl towards the palm, allowing baby to grasp objects or toys. It's more of an unrefined movement.

Around 9 to 10 months, but sometimes up to 12 months, your baby will start to develop a pincer grasp. This is when coordination between finger and thumb starts. It's also when you might be graced with the joy of comfort pinching – meaning the pincer grasp may come out not just around food, but also around your neck, boobs and underarm. Such a treat!

By using just the finger and thumb together, your baby will be able to pick up smaller objects, refining their motor skills. These movements are useful later for tasks such as holding a pencil, doing up buttons and using zips. Your baby will gradually improve the pincer grasp over a period of time, until they become experts.

HOW TO WEAN

You may have heard of baby-led weaning (BLW) or spoon-feeding and feel as though you need to pick one – but you don't have to choose one over the other. In fact, nutritionists and dieticians, supported by research, now encourage 'the best of both' approach. There's no evidence that combining approaches will confuse your baby or encourage choking. By offering both methods, your baby gets to explore a variety of feeding styles. The key is to do what feels right for you and your family, and be led by your baby's hunger and fullness cues. This is also known as 'responsive feeding'. Later in your baby's weaning journey, this means allowing your child to leave food when they are full and eat more at their request, and avoiding saying things like 'Just one more bite' or encouraging them to clear their plate.

HOW DO BABIES TASTE FOOD BEFORE THEY'RE BORN?

Babies are exposed to tastes way before they start weaning – flavours can transmit to amniotic fluid and breast milk. The 'carrot juice experiment' involved mums who drank carrot juice in pregnancy and the first two months of breastfeeding. Babies who were exposed to carrot juice during pregnancy and breastfeeding liked carrot-flavoured food cereal more than those who were not. Babies therefore have already experienced taste in utero and via breast milk.

After establishing your baby is ready to start solids, the next question on parents' minds is what to introduce first. In short, you can start weaning with single vegetables – try blended, mashed or soft-cooked sticks of parsnip, broccoli, potato, yam, sweet potato, carrot, apple or pear.

For many years, this was quite a regimented area and mothers/grandmothers of today's parents will have been given set advice. A lot of babies were weaned using 'baby rice', either homemade or from a packet. Then they would be introduced to mashed or puréed fruits, then vegetables. There were some varieties of jars of weaning food that are still available today (with a lot of choice and organic options added). Babies are hardwired to detect sweetness and to like it, and are therefore vulnerable to overconsumption of sweet food. That said, there is a lot we still do not know about early nutrition and taste.

Introducing more bitter and savoury flavours early on could help to develop your baby's taste preferences and set them up for a life of accepting different foods and flavours. Research suggests that the period of six to nine months is when babies are most accepting of new foods (referred to as the 'window of opportunity'). Repeated early exposure to vegetables builds on familiarity and acceptance. The research demonstrates that this approach can have a positive impact on vegetable intake. It's not guaranteed, nor is it the only way, but it's a consideration. Even if you do opt for a vegetable-led approach, it's possible that by the toddler phase they will still prefer sweet foods.

Why veg? Here are some compelling reasons:

- Vegetables are part of a balanced diet.
- They provide a source of fibre, an array of vitamins (including vitamins C and A), potassium and folate and minerals.
- Vegetables help to protect against health conditions, including obesity, cardiovascular disease and type 2 diabetes.

VEGGIE AND VEGAN FAMILIES

These dietary choices have hit record-level highs in recent years. Veganism wasn't at all popular ten years ago, whereas now it's very common and you can easily find many vegan alternatives to popular foods. There's also, yet again, a lot of conflicting advice out there, with some saying being vegan is a healthier lifestyle choice and others strongly disagreeing.

In short, I'm not qualified to provide you with in-depth nutritional advice, but I do think, although made complicated, it's rather simple.

Whole foods offer the best nutrition for the human body, processed foods do not. There are many alternatives to meat and dairy, but it's certainly worth looking at what those alternatives contain and whether or not they are a healthy option for you and your family. If your baby is being brought up veggie or vegan it's absolutely vital you understand the essential nutrients they need. For example, babies who have a vegan diet, which doesn't include dairy or eggs, need a supplement containing vitamin B12, or foods fortified with B12. Ask a health professional for advice.

What is recommended – and may seem counterintuitive – is to introduce potential allergens before 12 months of age, ideally at around six months. So that you can identify a reaction, it is best to introduce foods that can trigger allergic reactions one at a time. These are usually:

- cow's milk (in cooking or mixed with food)
- nuts and seeds (serve them crushed or ground)
- eggs (eggs without a Red Lion stamp should not be eaten raw or lightly cooked)
- foods that contain gluten, including wheat, barley and rye
- soya
- shellfish (don't serve raw or lightly cooked)
- fish

FOODS TO AVOID

Never offer the below foods whole as these could pose a choking hazard:

- grapes
- cherries
- nuts
- berries
- cherry tomatoes
- olives
- large pieces of fruit

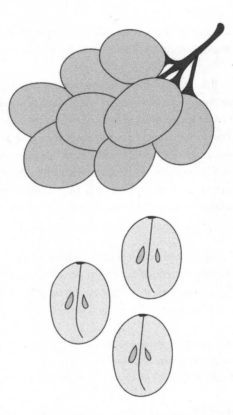

Small foods that present a choking hazard should be sliced into smaller pieces. Round fruits such as grapes, berries and cherry tomatoes should be sliced into quarters vertically and crushed. Nuts should be crushed, ground or served as nut butter.

The NHS also states that it's important not to offer babies and young children salt or salty foods (which includes bacon and sausages); sugar or sugary snacks; foods high in saturated fats; mould-ripened or blue-veined soft cheeses, ripened goat's milk cheese or cheeses made from unpasteurised milk; raw or lightly cooked eggs; rice drinks; raw jelly cubes; raw shellfish; or fish high in mercury, such as shark, marlin or swordfish.

Note: Occasionally, honey contains bacteria that can produce toxins in a baby's intestines, leading to infant botulism, which is a very serious illness. Therefore it is not recommended for babies under one to eat honey.

Charlotte Stirling-Reed is an award-winning baby and child nutritionist, mum to two young children, and *Sunday Times* bestselling author of *How to Wean Your Baby*. Here she has shared some tips on weaning your baby:

- Try not to have huge expectations – all babies take to weaning very differently and that's okay. Let them lead.
- Don't feel like you have to choose between baby-led weaning and purées/mashed food – a mix of both is fine.
- When it comes to finger foods, offer stick-shaped pieces of food (about the size of an adult's finger).
- Start with one meal a day initially and offer a single taste of something, like soft-cooked or puréed veggies, at that meal.
- Vary what you offer day to day to allow your baby to get used to a variety of new tastes and flavours early on.
- Remember it takes time to develop the skills needed to eat, so have patience and give them plenty of practice with finger foods and/or a spoon.
- Eat with them as this is the best way for them to learn to eat. It makes those mealtimes much more enjoyable for them too.
- Start building on that variety as your baby gets confident with eating and try to gradually move them on to more complex textures and similar meals to your family meals, without any sugar or salt.

> Charlotte Stirling-Reed, baby and child nutritionist

If you were nervous about weaning, I really hope this section has helped. A quote from my good friend, a mum of two little girls, may also help take the edge off your worries:

'The first time I did everything, and I mean everything, by the book. But when the second one came along, I just didn't have the same time or energy for it. I'll be honest, weaning for her meant mashing a banana and saying, "That's it, you're weaned!"'

> Michelle, mum of two

Try not to put too much pressure on yourself to get everything right and just explore with your baby. Be guided by them and try to enjoy this new phase if you can. A heads-up, though, one thing you may have more difficulty enjoying are their new poos, even more so if you are breastfeeding. Their poo goes from smelling sweet (and, I might add, rather pleasant) to real poo, as digested food passes through their bowels. I wish I had something positive to follow this up with, but I don't. In fact, the smell of their poo seems to gradually get worse and worse – a nappy bin may help to contain the pong.

GUT HEALTH FOR BABIES

The human body hosts millions of microorganisms (a.k.a. microbiota) that live on and inside us. These microorganisms interact with our own human cells and influence our health in many ways – throughout our lifetime. The 'microbiome' influences the immune system, endocrine system – where hormones are released – and neural pathways. There are a wide variety of microorganisms flourishing on the skin, in the mouth and in the genital tract, but what about those in the gut? Those are the most abundant and diverse. You have a whole other world living inside you.

Gut health is a very popular topic nowadays, as we are becoming more aware of how important it is to have a varied diet to help keep our gut healthy. Our gut produces healthy bacteria called flora. It takes a while for your baby to build up the flora, so it is worth understanding a little more about how to support this important process.

It's not just food that supports the colonisation of the gut. There are some other factors that can aid this process. An interesting study found there is a difference in the composition of bacteria for babies born via C-section compared to vaginal birth. As babies pass through the birth canal, they are exposed to billions of bacteria that are then transferred into the baby's body, gut and skin, training their immune system. You may (or may not) have heard of 'vaginal seeding', where mums rub vaginal fluid across the newborn baby's mouth and nose to mimic this if a baby is born via C-section. Breastfeeding also plays a significant role in boosting a baby's microbiome. So much so that research has revealed there is very little difference in gut health in babies born via C-section if breastfed for six months after birth. If you are bottle-feeding, please don't worry – you can support your baby's gut microbiome with probiotics. I currently use Baba West, which have a great range available. Also consider the formula milk you're giving and research the brand's ingredients. Many do include pre- and probiotics.

The skin microbiome also plays a role in overall health. Delaying your baby's first bath and using only water if you do choose to bathe them within the first month can support the body in building natural skin barriers and allow the skin microbiome to flourish (see pages 153–4 for more on bath time). Washing a baby with soap will likely interfere with this. Furthermore, having skin-to-skin exposes your baby to billions more bacteria, once again training and supporting the colonisation of gut bacteria. There is also some research into how pets (especially dogs) support gut health by leading to a more diverse microbiome.

Antibiotic exposure also affects the microbiome so it's always advisable only ever to give your baby antibiotics if absolutely necessary, especially within the first year of life. Research has shown that probiotic supplements may lessen the impact of antibiotics on a baby's gut microbiome, so this is worth discussing with your GP.

Your baby's personality

WE ALL HAVE different personalities; that's the beauty of being human, isn't it? We can learn from each other's ideas and understand more about human behaviour or our role within our society.

By nine months your baby's personality will likely be clear to see. They may display signs of an extrovert by being playful or inquisitive without shyness. They may be very happy exploring the world without you holding them or even being close to them. Or perhaps they are slightly more cautiously curious, preferring you to remain close by or to hold them while they explore.

Sometimes our baby's personalities and preferences can take us by surprise. We may therefore need to adjust our own expectations and adapt to them, for example, by choosing activities that best suit their temperament so they feel secure and safe. Providing reassurance and understanding of their needs builds on the trust and bond you have together. It may be tempting to encourage or even push them out of their comfort zone in order to learn how to cope, but most experts and child psychologists agree that it's best to support their individuality, letting them take the lead on what they're comfortable with. Once again, though, you know your baby better than anyone and you'll know the best way to nurture them.

HONESTY BOX

Georgie was a force to be reckoned with. She knows what she wants and can be very determined. I couldn't believe my eyes when I took her to baby soft play. She would pretty much ignore me. She wanted to explore in her own way and was happy to exclude me. At times I felt rejected by her and it was embarrassing when I would try to pick her up and she would scream and squirm away from me, as though I was a stranger. At home she would behave in the opposite way – she wanted all my attention and for me to carry her everywhere, showing great interest in what I was doing. That used to frustrate me sometimes – it was as though I had a different baby inside the house to outside. It took a while but I learnt to accept that about her; she wasn't excluding or rejecting me, she was confident, excited and just happy to explore on her own in new environments.

Comments from people around you, usually well-meaning family, can cause you to question your baby's behaviour. The most common remarks are: 'That baby's got you wrapped around their little finger' and, 'You're spoiling them and holding them too much.' Babies can sometimes be unfairly branded as manipulative. This simply isn't true – babies are not manipulative; they do not have the mental capacity to be. Although not a blank slate and far more capable than many researchers thought not so long ago, babies don't have the skills to think ahead about how to behave in order to achieve effect. Not yet anyhow. This is due to their immature brain.

An area of the brain called the pre-frontal cortex is where cognitive (thinking) skills are controlled. This complex region of the brain controls high-functioning abilities and social behaviour – almost like a 'personality centre'. This is the very last part of our brains to develop. On average it takes *approximately* 20 years to fully mature – depending on the person. What we can safely say is that a baby under the age of one does not have the mental capacity to display manipulative behaviour. At this young age, they act more impulsively. Babies communicate needs because they are genuine needs. From your perspective, you might want to prevent them from learning that a particular behaviour gets them what they want. This is something parents will debate. One parent may want to implement rules or boundaries, teaching a baby early on about things they need to accept, and another may not want to, instead believing that a young baby should have as many of their needs met as possible. This is a personal choice, but it's always important to remember the capability of a baby, alongside focusing on what feels instinctive to you.

'My partner and I really struggled with our views on parenting. She was so soft on our daughter and hardly ever told her off, instead she would always have an excuse for our daughter's behaviour. I found this hard because I didn't want to raise a bratty child who lacked respect for her parents. My partner wouldn't budge and kept telling me that I was wrong to want to discipline her a bit more. She would say she doesn't need it, she just needs love and validation. Honestly I thought it was such non-sense, all this emotional "validation", and believed people need to get a backbone. But I was wrong. Our daughter is so confident and she's not the brat I thought she would be. She certainly has her moments, but she's very loving and so sweet with other children. I am so proud of her. I do still think my partner is too soft and I have to set the rules. But it is a bal-ance, and I do think it's been good for our daughter to experience our different parenting styles.'

Anonymous, dad of one

Whatever your baby's personality, nurturing their nature and getting to know them as a person judgement-free is not always easy. But by embracing their traits you may find you develop a new skill set and teach them about self-compassion along the way. One of the biggest strengths in life is knowing yourself and being okay with that. By leading the way and letting them know that their nature is a beautiful one, you'll support them to have a good relation-ship with themselves and feel secure in who *they* are, potentially enabling them to be less inclined to people-please or go along with what others want them to do rather than doing what they want. Again, there are never any guarantees with how our children will turn out, and no parent is perfect, but these little messages you send and instil can support them overall and lead to the lifelong strength of being comfortable with themselves.

CARRYING YOUR BABY

~~~~

It's common for parents to carry younger babies, but not so much by the time they approach nine months. Carrying is still a great option, though, if you are happy to and they haven't become too heavy for you. Most babies are very happy to be carried at this age rather than be in a pram. They relish being out in the world and at your height they can enjoy a different perspective. I used to find using a baby carrier or sling very practical when I was getting on and off trains. There's no need to worry about asking for help with a buggy or hanging around waiting for lifts. Personally, I found it much easier to man-oeuvre. This isn't the case for everyone and some mums prefer the extra space to pop their bits and bobs under the buggy. Depending on where you are off to and your lifestyle, using a combination of the two may be helpful.

'By six to nine months it might be time to change things around or try a new carrier/sling. Look for them to be supported in a squat position, which is typically more comfortable for the wearer as it takes more of the baby's weight rather than their legs dangling down.'

Zoë, babywearing educational consultant, The Sling Consultancy

Illness

AT SOME POINT within the first year of life it is more than likely your baby will develop symptoms of an infection. There are four types of infections: viral, bacterial, fungal and parasitic. The common cold, stomach bugs or upper respiratory infections are all very common and are usually caused by a virus. If this is the case, antibiotics will not effectively treat the illness. By taking antibiotics for a viral illness, you could cause your baby more harm than good. Antibiotic resistance is a serious issue due to overuse in recent years.

Both the NHS and health organisations across the world are trying to reduce the use of antibiotics, especially for health problems that are not serious. For example, antibiotics are no longer routinely used to treat:

- chest infections
- ear infections in children
- sore throats

I hope the information below offers the help and support you need when your baby is unwell. However, as always, if you are concerned about your child's health, please consult your healthcare professional.

THE MOST COMMON CONDITIONS FOR BABIES UNDER ONE

The most common illness is a viral one. There are lots of different viruses and often there will be a wave of a particular strain of virus for a few weeks then it will calm down. The time of year also influences the viruses that are lurking around. With younger babies, viruses are better able to spread, which is why a respiratory infection or cold can then become an ear infection.

Symptoms do vary but commonly include things you're likely already aware of, such as:

- fever
- cold symptoms such as a runny nose and/or cough
- rashes – these can look different, from small red dots to larger patches of flushed skin or little pimples containing fluid on hands and feet and in the mouth
- vomiting
- more watery/softer poos
- tiredness
- change in mood, such as irritability or being clingy

TOP TIPS FOR HOME MANAGEMENT

With viral illnesses, it's important to know there isn't a pharmaceutical treatment, certainly not antibiotics. As we've just seen above, they do not work for viral infections and overuse of them is a global issue, so it's great to be aware of this as a parent. Antibiotics are generally prescribed for bacterial infections, or they can be used ahead of a procedure to prevent bacterial infection.

Your baby's little body is doing a great job of building an immune system, which is a vital part of human health. Although it's hard seeing your child battle with a virus, it's important to know how good the body is at clearing infection and support the body to do so. Take a look below at some further tips on this, which have been put together with the help of paediatrician Dr Richard Daniels.

Preventing dehydration

The younger the child, the faster they can become dehydrated. This is often more dangerous than the illness itself and so needs to be monitored. There are two simple measures to make sure the child is not getting overly dehydrated: what goes in, and what comes out.

Children may not want to eat or drink when unwell, especially if it is painful to swallow. This is completely normal. Almost forget about food – let them eat whatever they'll accept and do not stress about weight loss or nutrition; they'll catch up as soon as they feel better. Offer lots of fluids: milk is absolutely fine, but you can also offer cool, boiled water with a sachet of oral rehydration solution mixed in (Dioralyte is one brand name, but there are others), which can be mixed with a little bit of cordial or fruit juice to tempt the child to drink. **Consult a doctor or pharmacist before administering this**, and do not use in babies under three months. Little and often is a really good technique if they refuse to drink normally – you can use a medication syringe to give 5ml sips regularly.

Monitoring wet nappies is a must and helps you determine how well hydrated they are. If they are drinking less, the body will try to conserve fluid, so they will pass less urine. This can present as fewer wet nappies than usual, or little wees.

Overall, you should be aiming for about half of what they would usually drink and about half of the amount of urine they would usually pass to keep them safe until the illness is over. This is a rough guide – you do not need to get out the measuring jug! Always speak to a doctor if you are concerned.

Symptom control

Helping your baby control symptoms won't clear an infection, but it will make them feel a bit better. This means they are more likely to drink as outlined above.

Having a fever is not a problem in itself. It is part of the body's natural response to having an infection and actually helps the immune system fight infection. You may not need to treat a temperature or give them anything. If they are hot and happy, then you can monitor the rest of their symptoms (if any) and then decide whether or not they need medication. There's a great saying, 'Treat the child not the fever.' First always look at how your baby is behaving before reaching to treat them.

Fever and pain can be treated with medications that you can buy over the counter without a prescription. Paracetamol and ibuprofen both come in child-friendly formulations as a sugar-free flavoured syrup. It is usually safe to give a dose of paracetamol and then a dose of ibuprofen a few hours later, and then a dose of paracetamol a few hours after that, according to instructions. This means that they always have a dose of something in their system to keep the symptoms under control.

Under no circumstances should you give a child aspirin without the approval of a doctor. Aspirin can be dangerous for children.

For sore throats, you can get a numbing spray for the back of the throat. This is really effective, especially in getting a child to drink, but can only be given by a pharmacist or doctor. You can also buy cough syrups for children. They soothe the back of the throat, too, but do not work for as long as the spray.

Cold compresses are not recommended as they may make a child cold, which causes a new problem.

You should not give anything to a child under three months. It's best to get your baby seen by a medical professional as soon as possible if you have any concerns at this age. Many doctors are really cautious with what they recommend for babies under three months.

Avoid the obviously unwell

This is an obvious one, but, where possible, keep away from people who are unwell themselves, especially with newborn babies. What can be a mild illness for an adult can be a nasty illness for a small child. On that note, always ask visitors to wash their hands before cuddling your baby!

OTHER COMMON ILLNESSES

~~~~

Other common issues in babies and young children include skin rashes, such as eczema, reflux (see pages 122–4) and constipation. These are all unrelated to viruses but may cause similar concerns for parents.

Skin rashes

Two of the most common rashes are nappy rash and eczema. Nappy rash is caused by moisture being held against the skin by the nappy. This causes the skin to become inflamed and can progress to have the skin break down, or an infection find its way in.

To prevent nappy rash, you need to protect the skin from moisture, to let it dry out and heal. Try to change the nappy as frequently as possible to reduce the time the baby's skin spends in contact with a wet nappy pad, and, if possible, have plenty of nappy-free time to support the skin to dry. Generously apply a barrier cream after cleaning as it sits as a physical block on the skin. If the rash is not improving, then there may be a fungal infection on the skin requiring another cream. This can often be provided by your pharmacist.

Eczema presents as red blotchy patches that can look quite angry. The skin is dry and may crack. Often eczema is a condition that runs in the family.

Treatment initially is with moisturiser, or emollient, which can be bought over the counter without a prescription. There are several types to choose from – some are more greasy than others, which are more effective but also more messy. You can use a soap substitute to wash your child, as soap often dries out the skin further. Active patches that have flared might need a steroid cream for a few days until the inflammation resolves. This needs to be given by a pharmacist or doctor.

Most skin rashes will self-resolve. But baby skin is much more sensitive than adult skin, meaning rashes appear frequently.

Constipation

Constipation is seen a lot in babies, especially around the time they start weaning. They tend to poo less frequently as they get older and a problem usually occurs when they're in pain and then don't want to go. Constipation is usually diagnosed if a baby has stomach pain, fewer than three motions a week with hard stools or, conversely, diarrhoea.

Constipation is really common and may come and go. There are lifestyle and medication treatment options. Lifestyle changes include a balanced diet containing natural fibres, such as those found in wholemeal foods, fruit and vegetables, and plenty of water to drink.

Laxatives are the mainstay of medical treatment. These can be used to clear out hard stools and then to maintain softer stools going forward. If you think your baby needs laxatives, make an appointment to see a doctor as these can only be provided on prescription.

WHEN SHOULD I SEEK HELP?

Dr Richard Daniels advises that this depends on age. Newborn babies need to be seen by a healthcare professional much earlier than a big, strapping 11-month-old.

As above, he always advises parents to bring any baby under the age of three months to be seen by a paediatrician if they have a temperature over 38°C. Under three months, the immune system is not as well developed and the risk of serious illness is increased. The important thing to consider for this age group is how the baby is behaving. Doctors look for a few things here:

- How is the child breathing?
- How is the child drinking?
- How are the child's nappies?
- How is the child behaving?

Of course, if you are concerned at any point, you can always seek advice from a healthcare professional.

'Reassuring worried parents that their child is all right is one of my favourite parts of my job, and I'd rather see 1,000 people and send them all home than have someone stay away for fear of "wasting my time" and the child getting worse. You are not wasting our time – that is what we are here for.'

Dr Richard Daniels, paediatrician

LOOKING AFTER YOURSELF AS WELL AS YOUR BABY

Initially, the thought of your baby becoming unwell may worry you. As they get bigger and stronger it is likely the more pressing issue you'll have to manage is the impact this has on you. When your little one is ill, they often don't sleep as well. They may be up coughing throughout the night, crying and being irritable during the day. To top it off, you'll likely catch whatever it is they've got. Illness can be really hard for you too, mama. If you're caring for your baby, loving and soothing them, you deserve that too. Which brings us on to . . .

Mama self-care

LOOKING AFTER YOURSELF is part of looking after your baby. You aren't able to be the best version of yourself if you don't practise basic self-care. When I say self-care, you're possibly picturing a bath with rose petals or doing an hour's yoga session. Those things can be, if you have got the time, but for mums with young babies self-care often means meeting your basic human needs, like eating, drinking enough water, getting some exercise, and paying attention to pain or discomfort in your body. The more you ignore warning signs, the worse they become. For example, dehydration doesn't go away and it can make you feel awful and cause long-term health complications, yet it's so easily avoided when you instil basic self-care into your life.

'My resentment towards my husband and his lifestyle started during pregnancy. I would kiss my husband goodbye as he headed off out on a Saturday night with the boys, full of FOMO and resentment. It's strange because I really was happy to be pregnant but I did find it hard to let go of my old life and accept the transformation – which began suddenly. The longing for my old life disappeared almost immediately after birth as I was on a real oxytocin high, but at around four months after birth it came back with a vengeance. I just wanted my freedom, to have a lie-in, have a day off and to leave the house without a care in the world. At times, I felt selfish for missing my old life but came to realise more recently that I need to be compassionate towards myself about this because it is hard to give up so much of yourself and your comforts.'

Anonymous, mum of one

HONESTY BOX

I looked after myself pretty well in the fourth trimester – there was room for improvement, but I didn't do too badly. However, by the time Georgie was six months old I was exhausted, empty, thirsty, unhealthy, sluggish and lacked self-compassion. It's sad to admit, but I watched myself deteriorate between six and ten months. Sleep deprivation was mainly to blame, but that led to a cascade of issues and a lack of basic self-care. I would hold a wee in during the night for many hours in fear of waking Georgie up. One night my bladder felt like it was about to rupture before I had no choice but to take the risk and prioritise my basic need to urinate. I'd force myself out to soft play without eating or drinking a full glass of water. Because *she* needed it. I would have a constant narration of her day running in my mind, including all the things she might need or feel: had she had enough to eat? Had I stimulated her enough or given her enough attention? Totally forgetting what I needed, which wasn't a strong coffee that had gone cold because I'd rushed around with the hoover cleaning up after her food fight with the floor, or shoving a chocolate bar in my face to give me a boost. What I really needed was to do a few things from the list below.

YOUR NEEDS MATTER

Here are a few things to help you look after yourself:

- Reach out to a friend or family member for physical support or to verbally offload.
- Go to bed as early as possible.
- Put your phone on aeroplane mode before bed and leave it out of reach – ideally in another room.
- Drink calming herbal teas and increase your water intake.
- Put a boundary in place – this could be reducing time spent on someone or something, like a draining friend or social media.
- Change your bed sheets and pop some lavender oil on the pillows.
- Listen to your favourite music or put on a podcast.
- Take a long shower or bath, wash your hair, and moisturise when you get out.

- Batch-cook, if you've got it in you, so you have hearty meals ready to reheat for the next few days – lentil soup can be a good one, as are Bolognese, ratatouille and stews.
- Write down or bring to mind three things you are grateful for every morning or evening. These can be simple, like your warm comfy bed, your breakfast or running water.
- Take deep breaths in through the nose and out through your mouth as often in the day as you can.
- Repeat 'I let go of what I cannot control and focus on what I can' and 'This too shall pass.'
- Attend a local yoga class – the stretching and breathing are beneficial to your body and mind.
- Notice what's going on with your body, how you feel, validate those feelings and say something kind to yourself like, 'This is a lot to manage, you're doing amazing!'
- Take vitamins or probiotics, such as vitamins C, D, iron and fermented foods like kimchi.
- Before you go to bed, write down three things that are essential for the following day – ignore any other buzzing in your mind. You have your focus and that's all you can manage at the moment.
- Read this section a few times.

Eventually, carving out time for myself and prioritising my needs saw a huge shift in my health and happiness – alongside asking Andy to get up two nights a week with Georgie. You don't have to put yourself through months of self-neglect to get to a place of understanding and accepting how much *your* needs really matter. Managing mum life like that is not sustainable and I wish more than anything I'd taken better care of my needs during that time. You deserve basic self-care at the very least – that's a fact. Once you've implemented the basics you can start to build on your needs when you're ready. I now go to yoga, the gym, see a physiotherapist, and once a week I take an hour out for myself to do something I enjoy. I even go for tapas an hour before I collect Georgie from nursery on a Thursday – because I deserve it and the glass of red to wash it down. Not one part of me feels guilt for that because I'm proud to say I look after myself. It may take time for you to be able to build up to that point, but if you can get there, I promise you something, mama, you won't regret it.

TIRED GAMES

When you're tired or getting over an illness, it can be really hard to think of ways to entertain your baby. Here are a few ideas I found helpful:

- Have a bath together or watch them play in the bath safely. Get yourself something comfy to sit on rather than leaning over the bath. We use a little fold-up stool.
- Place a big tablecloth on the kitchen floor and (safely) put on it bowls of dry rice, pasta, lentils, water or whatever else you have around that's safe in the presence of your baby. Sit nearby with a cuppa and watch. Be mindful whatever you put down will likely end up in their mouth.
- Rip up paper or tissue – most babies love this.
- Put a bubble machine on (if you have one).
- Lie on the floor with them and play peek-a-boo. When they get bored, start rolling – it works!
- Create a treasure box. Put safe items they don't usually play with, like keys, silver spoons, old loyalty cards, etc., in a box and watch them explore. Change the items up for the next time you need to get the box out.

HONESTY BOX

Georgie had her first sleepover at our house with my good friend and her two girls. In the morning I made sure they all had a drink and was faffing around, putting toys away from the night before, chucking the leftovers in the bin. My friend came down and I carried on, while chatting to her. After a few minutes she said, 'Can I put the kettle on?' I realised I had totally forgotten to offer her a drink. I made us a hot drink and, as I passed it to her, she said, 'Why don't you come and sit down to have that?' Our kids were playing happily and watching TV so I sat down for about three minutes and then said, 'Right, shall I start making them breakfast?' She looked at me lovingly and replied, 'Let's just drink this before the chaos of the day begins; they're happy playing.' That stuck with me and I still hear her voice now when I find myself starting unnecessary tasks that no one is prompting me to do.

Self-care is not selfish. Taking care of yourself looks different for different people and can even look different for you on different days. Try to tune in to yourself and identify what you need to best care for yourself. If you wait for the big moments, holidays or whole evenings out, you'll miss out on all the little things you can do daily that add up to your needs being met and you feeling better. And I hope the tired games help!

KEY POINTS

- Babies do things at different times and have different personalities. It's best to parent their individuality rather than your expectations.
- Weaning is a whole new exciting but potentially scary phase. Remember, we all learnt to eat and your baby will get the hang of it eventually.
- Look for the physical signs your baby is ready to wean and avoid advice from outsiders pushing you to wean early.
- Dealing with your baby's first illness, coughs and colds can be taxing for you – remember to look after yourself too.
- Tune in to yourself and notice your needs. If you wait for the big things, like a holiday or date night, you may miss out on all the little things you can be doing for yourself daily.
- You're superwoman.

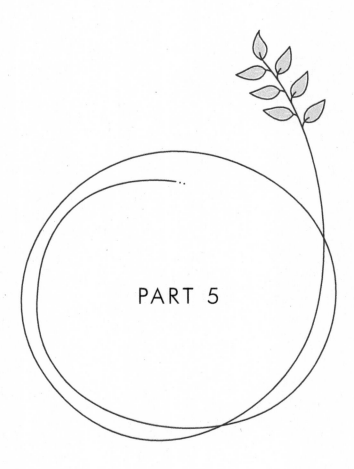

PART 5

Nine to Twelve

Months

~~~~~

Welcome to the final section, where we will cover those last few months before your baby's first birthday! Massive congratulations to you, mama, you really have done an incredible job of raising the future and getting through the first year – packed with milestones and dramatic ups and downs.

In this last section we will start off by exploring your baby's world and how you can support their growth and development. We'll then cover some of the things you may be experiencing or planning, like going back to work, and finish up on some more self-care tips and reminders to take with you on your onward journey.

What to expect

WHEN YOUR BABY is around the age of one, you should have an appointment with your health visitor for their 10–12-month review. You may be asked to fill in the 12-month ASQ-3 (Ages & Stages Questionnaire) ahead of the appointment. Don't worry if you can't or aren't sure as your health visitor will do this with you. The one-year page in their red book also highlights the new skills you may spot emerging at this age.

The 10–12-month review is an opportunity for you and a healthcare professional to have a look at your baby's progress. Your health visitor or nurse will likely discuss the following with you:

- healthy eating
- dental health
- keeping the home safe
- speech and language advice
- sleep
- what do to if your baby becomes unwell
- any concerns/questions you have

Some mums have expressed their fear around this check and admitted to feeling as though it's an assessment of their parenting. This really isn't the case; it's a shared conversation between you and the health visitor. They simply want to support you and answer any questions you have. There's nothing at all to worry about, you've done amazingly well.

'There's been quite a lot of negative feedback about the questionnaire because it is a tick-box exercise and we may see a lot of physical development that on paper might look like they're not quite hitting their milestones. Actually, when you're there with the child you can see them, they're doing so much stuff and they've got the strength to be able to do it and they're developing beautifully.'

Laura Smith, specialist community public health nurse (health visitor) Ebonie Chandraraj, specialist community public health nurse (health visitor) @gentlehealthvisitors

MESS

~~~~

You may notice that your baby loves to make a mess, pull things apart, bash things together and pour things all over the floor. Getting their little hands on a bag of lentils to throw across the floor is their version of throwing confetti at a wedding – the messier the better, with no consideration for who's doing the clearing-up. This is very normal and a healthy part of their development. As they get closer to one, or just after, you may notice they start doing the opposite – they like to put things back together and see how that works, or combine the two: destruct then reassemble. (Not always, though; they may stick with the destruction phase for some time – we were there for around two years!) They may also have a danger radar, for all the wrong reasons. If it's dangerous, they're drawn to it!

SPEECH AND BABBLING

~~~~

Although not a huge or particularly obvious difference, from 9–12 months you may see some progression in their speech. Your baby may copy sounds you make and love a game of peek-a-boo, perhaps copying words like 'boo'. Some babies do say their first word around one. Others don't say many words at all for a while after their first birthday. But they'll squeal or make noises responding in their own little way, which is all progress and communication. Georgie didn't say many words clearly until around 18 months. A lovely grandma I met in the park told me, 'They're either walkers or talkers,' and was utterly convinced by this. Some agree with the theory, others don't. In short, as we've already seen, babies all do different things at different times based on their personality and what they find most interesting about their world.

CLINGY

~~~

You may notice your baby has become particularly clingy again and wants to be carried around, even if they are mobile and able to get themselves from A to B. They may want to watch and be part of everything you do. If you're not doing much that interests them, they may try to entice you into a game or demand your attention in other ways. They usually want not only to be near you but on you and you can find yourself becoming a human climbing frame, which is far more interactive than anything else they can climb. You move, make noises and have various textures, like skin and hair. Getting an elbow to the boob is never fun, so do gently but firmly set your boundaries if you're not up for it.

OTHER BEHAVIOURAL CHANGES

~~~

Around the age of one you may start to get a glimpse of your baby's sense of humour. They can crack up laughing at the most random games or noises. A common one is paper being ripped as mentioned in the list of tired games (see page 199) – babies seem to love this and even find it funny, especially if you add the special-effect noises to go with it. They may be able to copy or pull funny faces themselves and be really pleased with this. Their cheeky and mischievous side may start to appear too, if it hasn't already. This can also be a challenging time as they may display behaviour that we view as unkind, such as pinching, biting or pulling hair. Although frustrating (and painful), your baby isn't trying to be mean or hurt you. They're curious, exploring and acting on impulse. They will grow out of this behaviour. I know it can be really tough if they attack another child. Your parenting style will support you to manage these tricky situations, but do bear in mind that they don't plan to cause harm or understand the damage they are capable of.

HONESTY BOX

I want to remind you that you don't have to prove yourself to anyone. Some days you won't have the energy for it – I've been there. I have not stopped Georgie from taking a toy off another child because I simply did not have the energy for it on that day. I can't always be the best version of myself, and there are times I need to sit and finish my hot drink rather than jump in every second she behaves in a way that's perceived to be 'inappropriate'. They're babies, they act like babies and that's okay. Many nurseries, unless a child is having pain inflicted or is at risk of danger, let the situation play out. Children learn from these interactions. They learn about themselves, their boundaries, the world, communication and more. You may not always be comfortable with their behaviour; it's challenging but, mostly, it's normal. So next time you're in and among the soft play madness and your baby acts 'inappropriately', take the pressure off. Do what you think is right, not what you think the other parent expects from you. The more I've taken that attitude into soft play, the more enjoyable it has been for me.

BUILDING ON KNOWLEDGE

You may start to see them handling their toys in different ways. They go from wanting not just to hold something but to see what they can do with it, wondering what happens if they press a button, for example. Or poke an object through a hole. Will it come out the other side? They're learning sequences and spotting patterns, which is a critical skill in adulthood. It's how we simulate situations. We do this all day, every day, using the laws of physics. Your baby may try a sequence they have seen, such as putting food on a plate, clapping at an appropriate time (usually for themselves upon completing a task) or putting their shoes near their feet. This is all so wonderful to see as they're making sense of their environment – what a lovely realisation it must be for them that life is not entirely random. Around this time your baby may also *begin* to understand categories and groups, such as round blocks in comparison with square, or the difference between humans and animals. Reading is a great way of helping babies to identify objects and categories, too.

THE NEED TO NAP

~~~

Babies will still nap for a while, usually until around the age of three or just before, some younger and some older. They will gradually drop naps as they grow. At this age, on average, they need around 11–14 hours of sleep in a 24-hour period, including naps.

CURIOSITY DRIVES LEARNING

~~~

Pierre-Yves Oudeyer, research director at the French Institute for Research in Computer Science and Automation (Inria) has an interest in how babies learn through curiosity. He decided to run a very interesting experiment which highlighted the importance of curiosity to the learning process. In summary, he concluded that being free to explore is the most efficient and quickest way to learn skills. So incentivising babies to solve specific problems may actually be counterproductive and it's best to let them be curious, to explore freely.

Reaction to action is part of learning and something we continue to learn throughout our lives. For babies, this learning is in its infancy and we need to nurture that, allowing them to knock things over (safety permitting) or drop objects. Observing this movement is part of learning the art of anticipation. As adults, the more we anticipate, the fewer mistakes we make. Understanding movement is really essential to a baby.

During the first year of life, babies go on an internal and external movement journey. They are constantly learning about their own bodies, what they are capable of already and how to progress. At the very same time they are learning about how the external world works too: how objects move, gain speed and are slowed down, for example. It's a magical time full of things they're naturally motivated to learn about. Many babies will relentlessly self-challenge and probe the boundaries of what they can do, pushing them to the next phase. They are very aware and intelligent in their own way, often taking parents by surprise as they suddenly leap forward to the next milestone.

As this all happens so fast you may miss parts of it – you're focused on keeping them safe, making sure they are fed, well-rested and stimulated. If you can, try to stop for little moments in the day to absorb what they're doing and take videos to look back on. Their world is expanding in front of your very eyes.

MOBILITY

~~~~

Some, but not all, babies will be mobile by 12 months, either crawling, bum-shuffling or taking their first steps. Some skip crawling entirely and go straight to walking. They often use you or furniture as props to pull themselves up and attempt to stand. All of a sudden it may seem as though your tiny baby is growing up and becoming more independent.

Georgie took her first steps at nine months and I could not let her leave my sight for a second – she was quick and had no sense of danger or fear. On average, I saved her life around 20 times a day, every day for months. It was an amazing time but also scary. I lived in fear of her hurting herself from the moment she opened her eyes every morning. Some days I was so exhausted I couldn't keep up with her – we had baby-proofed the house (see below), which took some pressure off, but when we left the house it was game on. I don't remember one time I took her out and felt relaxed; everything I attempted was interrupted – a conversation, a sandwich or a sip of coffee. That's not to say you won't be able to relax; maybe your baby is happy sitting on your lap and is entertained by looking rather than touching or grabbing dangerous things. Or maybe you have a Georgie character who has to reach for danger and keeps you on your toes at all times. They're all so different, but either way they are all a liability and you need to create safe environments for them to play and move around in.

BABY-PROOFING TIPS

Start with keeping dangerous objects or liquids out of reach or behind cupboard doors fitted with baby locks. You also need to rearrange the home and your habits to ensure they don't hurt themselves. Here are some things to consider for now:

- Make sure hot drinks are out of reach. It's easy for a baby to grab a hot drink in your hand or bump into a coffee table and knock over a mug.

- Keep electrical and other cables out of your baby's reach and tie up any cords, such as those on blinds. These can be very dangerous as babies love putting things around/over their head.
- Fit stair gates to stop your baby getting up or down the stairs.
- Make sure there aren't any sharp objects within your baby's reach. Razors are a common one, left on the side of the bath or in the shower.
- Keep a close eye on your baby around water. Small children can drown in less than 5cm of water. For the same reason, never leave your baby unattended in the bath.
- Keep domestic bleach, medications and other dangerous substances either way out of your baby's reach or in a baby-proofed cupboard.
- If cooking, ensure you use the hobs at the back of the stove and never leave handles in reach.
- Secure heavy furniture so they can't pull it over on to themselves.
- Cover sharp edges or corners.
- Lock windows or install restrictors.
- Get some door stoppers or catches to hold doors open so they can't trap their little fingers.

Hopefully this advice helps with planning, but remember, accidents do happen. You can do all the baby-proofing in the world, yet they may still take you by surprise and manage to hurt themselves somehow. Or you may forget about a particular danger one day. If this happens, please don't beat yourself up about it. Mistakes happen and you can only ever do your best.

'We were in a rush one day and I popped her in the buggy, grabbed the bags, snacks and, you know, the armour you take out with you. Rushed down the driveway reaching the kerb, tilted the pram forward and . . . BANG! She fell out and hit her head right on the pavement. I had forgotten to strap her in. I felt terrible. We sat on the side of the road and cried together as I pulled my phone out to call 111.'

Anonymous, mum of two

WORRIED ABOUT WALKING?

As we've already touched on, it's very easy to compare your baby to others and, if you see your friend's baby steady on their feet, you can naturally start to question why your baby isn't doing the same. All babies have their own inner timeline and that is normal for them. By comparing you may cause yourself unnecessary stress and worry. Next week they may get there, or next month. You're both doing great!

'Lots of children who don't walk till 15, 16, 17 months are perfectly healthy and well with no long-term problems. Often it depends on the bigger picture; for example, if there are other concerns with areas of development, or parents are worried that they aren't developing as they expect them to be. Crawling is a good indicator because you can see their strength, you can see they're using all their limbs equally. The vast majority of babies walk within the recommended timeframe.'

Laura Smith, specialist community public health nurse
(health visitor) Ebonie Chandraraj, specialist community public
health nurse (health visitor) @gentlehealthvisitors

DISCIPLINE

This word means different things to different people and depends on your culture and upbringing. In some cultures, it's very much acceptable to hit children, leaving marks and bruises. Here in the UK it is not, and parents can be prosecuted for this. Regardless of UK law and culture, hitting a baby under one is only ever going to cause them harm – physically and/or emotionally.

As your baby edges closer to one, they can begin to press your anger button more often, and controlling your own emotions can gradually become harder as they progress from a helpless baby to a slightly more aware toddler. In the moments you experience anger, frustration and despair, STOP. Put them in a safe place and take a moment – it's okay to create that separation when you need it.

HONESTY BOX

Once, when Georgie was 11 months old, she wouldn't nap. I remember it clearly because it got ugly. I was looking forward to her nap; we'd had a busy morning and she'd been up in the night a few times and been on and off the boob. I hadn't had a minute to myself in over 24 hours – not one minute. When she refused to nap after repeated attempts to settle her, I lost it. In an angry, exhausted haze I lost control of myself and shouted at her like I had never shouted before, then started hysterically crying and resorted to begging her to nap. Of course, she still refused. I needed to be away from her for a moment, so I left her safely in her cot and walked downstairs to the kitchen. I put my hand on my heart and took a few deep breaths, repeating, 'This too shall pass.' Always opt for time out if you can feel yourself about to lose it.

Putting your needs first

I WROTE THIS section and kept moving it from chapter to chapter, unable to identify the most timely place for it. Then I realised something – there is no set time. The timing of deciding you need to prioritise yourself varies significantly from person to person and depends on several factors – your approach, your baby's needs and their age. Overall, you should aim to put your needs first as often as possible, as early as possible. When I say 'needs', I mean your basic needs: to eat, drink, shower, go to the toilet and feel comfortable. It's hard because a newborn is so very reliant on you and there are many times when you need to prioritise them. Balancing your needs and theirs, as they grow and become more independent, is more of a juggling act and a trade-off.

Prioritisation doesn't have to be all or nothing, or one rule that's applied to all scenarios. Your choices should be fluid and flexible depending on your commitments and other factors you need to consider. Perhaps the lead-up to your period and feeling tried or fed up may mean you're not up for the stimulation of soft play. Or a bad night with several wakings has left you drained. You may then need the comfort of your home and entertainment for your little one indoors may well do for the morning. Then maybe a walk to the park in the afternoon, getting you both out in the fresh air, is enough for you on that day. There will always be compromises to be made and implementing these early on can set you up to have a better relationship with yourself and your baby.

Depression is an unbelievably common problem for new mums, leading to some particularly startling statistics on suicide in the UK. The largest population-based study to date found that 17.22 per cent of mothers globally suffered with PND, equating to millions of mothers every single year. The causes of depression are often multifactorial and there is rarely one solution to help manage or prevent it. But what I will say we do know is that a lot of depressed mums don't feel capable of doing 'the job' or feel good enough about themselves, which leads to self-sabotage and self-neglect. If you get into the habit of constantly ignoring your needs, it can be hard to see where these fit in further down the line. The cycle may therefore continue, leading you to a difficult place. Leaving you questioning: 'Is it okay to put myself first?' Which is exactly what happened to me . . .

HONESTY BOX

There have been a few occasions when I have really not wanted to do something but have forced myself – like breastfeed Georgie, aged almost two, and let her fiddle with my other nipple. This is very normal behaviour for breastfed babies, and it's done for comfort, contact and to help with milk let-down. The sensation was horrible, plus I'd had enough of the constant request for 'boobie' and it all got too much. I fed her reluctantly, thinking, 'It's my duty, maybe her molars are playing up again,' but as she was feeding the sensation and combination of her sucking and fiddling became more and more irritating. I had to take her off. She became angry with me but I explained, 'Mummy's feeling sore now,' and handed her to Andy. I then took myself off to our bedroom, cried and screamed into a pillow. I'd hit my boundary loud and clear. I could not give any more of myself. The screaming into a pillow wasn't just because her fiddling/feeding was irritating. It was the culmination of events leading up to this. I'd ignored my own needs so much for so long. I suddenly realised that I'm not a slave to her needs and it's not okay for me to feel high levels of discomfort to satisfy her anymore. She needed to learn that I have boundaries. This battle manifests itself in different ways for many mums, not just when it comes to feeding a toddler. In order to be the mother I would like to be (which looks different for everyone, and that's okay, whatever your version is) I had to start respecting my own needs. She too needed to learn to respect them. I wish someone had told me how to set boundaries and given me permission to say no.

Going back to work (or not)

WHATEVER YOU DECIDE to do regarding work is a very personal choice. Some mums want to take time out of their careers and would rather be with their children. Other mums really look forward to getting back to work. And some have a choice to work or not work. You may feel judged no matter what you do. Out of curiosity I posted a question box on Instagram about this and got hundreds of replies, many revealing judgements made about both working and stay-at-home mums. A number of mums reported that they had been asked, 'Do you work or are you just a housewife?' and others recounted family members' comments on them going back to work 'too soon'.

Mama, you do you, because it's not onlookers who will suffer the consequences if you don't. Of course, on occasion, those around you who love and care about you may question your choices with the intention of supporting you. But plain judgement? That's not helpful or something you should carry around with you.

If you are returning to work, you may feel a real mix of emotions and conflicting feelings as your mind plays out the reality of leaving your baby with someone else. You may be hanging on to every new thing your baby does and wishing you had more time off as your maternity leave comes to an end. Yet on the same day find yourself clock-watching until bedtime finally arrives.

The truth is, it's normal. All of the emotions – excitement, resentment, nervousness, guilt, doubt, happiness and relief. The need to protect them is overwhelming, especially when they are under one. Mum guilt will often find a way to creep in no matter what you do or who you leave them with. Picking up your job title and putting it back on has its own demands too. But for some mums, being focused on something other than their baby, and having adult conversations, can give them a break from the demands of motherhood.

NOT WANTING TO RETURN TO WORK

~~~~

When heading off for your mat leave you may have had a plan for what you were going to do after having your baby. Or maybe you weren't too sure. Some mums plan to return to work but, as their maternity leave draws to a close, they feel very unsure about going back. It can be such a tough decision and end up keeping you up at night more than your baby! To help you make a decision, write out a list of pros and cons. The only person who can decide is you and this may also be heavily guided by circumstances.

Deciding not to go back can be gut-wrenching and cause a lot of emotional distress, grief and confusion. You may find you hit a bit of an identity crisis. Your views on your work and home life are in plain sight and it can be hard to choose where you want to spend your time. We certainly do not have it easy here, mamas. As I've mentioned throughout the book, society does not value mothers in the way that it should, with some people referring or alluding to mat leave as a 'break', giving the impression that motherhood is easy and we sit drinking tea all day. This can add further weight to your decision, as it appears some, at times, don't view staying at home and raising children – namely, the hardest job in the world – as having the same value as going to work. Someone actually asked me what I did on mat leave, like it was a form of annual holiday and I'd be able to share all the fun I'd had. Seriously. They got a very sarcastic answer. Comments like 'Do you work or are you *just* a stay-at-home mum?' can really cut deep. Anyone who uses that kind of word-ing (although subtle, it tells you what they think) around motherhood and raising children is not a person you need to value in your life right now. That may sound harsh, but I'm here to support you and your decisions, so I'm not going to make excuses for someone who lacks appreciation for what you're doing. You are doing an incredible job of raising the future – keep shining!

Mums who plan to return to work out of necessity can feel heartbroken in the lead-up. If this is you, ensure you explore *all* options first. These days, there is usually more flexibility for mums returning to work than there used to be. Post-pandemic, working from home has also become a more feasible option, if your job role accommodates this. There are, of course, pros and cons to it all. Arrangements may need to be worked out and trialled before you commit yourself contractually. Remember, everything is negotiable prior to formal agreements, so do try to advocate for yourself and negotiate. The more con-fident you are in this the better – know your worth and be confident that your skill set is a great asset to the company.

It may be worth considering the following:

- The cost of childcare versus income generated (sometimes there's not a lot in it if you don't have free help).
- Reducing outgoings to make up for loss of income.
- Do you have any skills you could utilise as a freelancer?
- Career change that enables more flexibility, such as a sleep consultant, home beauty therapist or starting your own business. Common sense, but you'll need to factor in the time and cost it will take to build clients/ the business.
- Discussing extension of maternity leave with your employer or job-sharing.
- Discussing part-time hours with your employer.
- Are there any benefits you are entitled to?

Many new businesses are born while mums are on maternity leave. It can be scary starting up a business or being self-employed, but there are many benefits to this too. Including freedom.

WANTING TO RETURN TO WORK

As mentioned, even if you want to return to work you may question yourself or worry about how your baby will cope. My good friend Erika, who I met outside Georgie's nursery, works in a very senior role for one of the biggest companies in the world. She highly values her goals and professional working life, and has often offered me support when I've had a little cry in the car park.

Juggling has been really tough at times and I've been riddled with mum guilt. Deep down, I know Georgie is very happy at nursery. She has a network of friends, a lot of fun with messy play, baking biscuits, painting, playing games, singing, dressing up, and she's almost always happy to be dropped off. Sometimes she doesn't even look back to wave me off. I can't stimulate her the same way nursery can. As she's got older, she's built strong bonds with the other children and they run over shouting, 'Georgie!' when she arrives – it's so beautiful to see.

Me continuing to work is the best option for both of us. I am deeply passionate about my career and supporting mothers. I am allowed to be passionate about those things and love my daughter dearly. Whatever you choose in terms of childcare (see options in box below), you need to be comfortable with your decision and feel able to focus on your work. It's counterproductive and becomes stressful if you're in one place and thinking about another, wishing you were there, which is also the description of not being present in the moment. You'll naturally think about your baby a lot while you're away from them initially, but long-term you do need to be able to focus, distraction-free.

CHILDCARE OPTIONS

- Nursery: prices and opening hours vary, but usually a full day is 10–11 hours.
- Registered childminder: prices and opening hours vary.
- Family/friends: may be free or a cheaper option; set your own hours.
- Nanny: prices and hours usually negotiable.
- Live-in au pair: as above.
- Crèches: usually for an hour or so only.
- Pre-school: may only offer short days and often term-time only.

Tip: remember to check on the government website regarding benefits or credits you may be entitled to. This may save you hundreds every month!

For me nursery was the best option and where I felt most comfortable leaving Georgie. I had access to a special system where I could see photos and videos of her during the day, the building is secure, and I knew I wouldn't get calls unless I was really needed. All mums are different, so you may want to 'try on your future'. This is something I do all the time. I get the options clear in my mind and I vividly picture myself carrying them out. I visualise how I feel and what happens, then the decision tends to be made for me. Because this is imaginary, it won't always be accurate but it gets you in tune with your gut and can be a helpful tool if you need to make a decision. In the lead-up to your return to work, ensure your baby gets used to other people, whoever you trust. Leave them for short intervals and see how they get on. They may surprise you! This will also help during their settling in period with whoever you leave them with.

If you're experiencing struggles with leaving your baby, but are confident working is what you want to do, Erika may be able to offer you some words of wisdom too:

'Keep in mind that your work colleagues might also be parents, so don't feel guilty if you have to miss a meeting or finish earlier because you need to rush back to your baby. People understand that our biggest commitment is our little one.

Sometimes it's hard, but don't bring work-related stress back home. Giving quality time to your kid is the most important thing, so when you are not at work, plan happy/uplifting activities with your baby – play dates, park time, movie time, etc. These create strong bonds and make little ones feel loved and attended to.

At the beginning it can be really hard to leave your baby. However, you need to remember that you are also a professional and you worked hard to be where you are in your career. Also, before you can imagine, your kid will be at school, so taking care of your professional life is important and will probably make you feel good as well as updated.'

Erika, mum of one, pregnant with baby number two

Upon returning to work, be aware of burnout. A 2018 study published by the Business Performance Innovation Network found that 63 per cent of parents who work outside the home have experienced some form of parental burnout. As much as you can, find little ways to nurture and replenish your body and mind. Exercise, even if it's just going for a quick walk on your lunch break, can help aid blood flow and ease the stress of work. Remember to also use any employee benefits – if you have them.

Companies have a responsibility to provide equitable and appropriate work environments, alongside private pumping areas, job-sharing options and subsidised childcare. Some companies are really on top of their game when it comes to supporting new parents and even go above and beyond the basic requirements. And some are lagging behind. The more pressure we apply collectively, the quicker they'll catch up.

I am no careers advisor, but my good friend Helen Tupper is, and she's got some tips for mums who aren't happy in their current job but want to work:

'I've never felt my career has been compromised by being a parent. In fact, it's the opposite. I have more empathy for others, better boundaries for myself and a more balanced perspective on how work contributes to my life. This has been better for the relationships I've built at work and much better for my business too. Some important things have contributed: flexible employment, support with childcare (both from family and paid-for childcare) and prioritising my health so I can do my best when my sleep is broken and when it feels like there are too many things to do in a day. It's not always easy and sometimes you have to make tough choices, but your career doesn't have to be compromised by being a parent.'

Helen Tupper, podcaster, co-author of *The Squiggly Career* and CEO of Amazing If

HANDING YOUR CHILD OVER

It's so important to have a think about your plans and get in early doors. Calling upon family and friends may be an option you want to explore and figure out how this could work. Childminders usually have more availability, but nurseries often have ridiculously long waiting lists. I did not know quite how long until, five months before I was due to return to work, I called a nursery and asked about visiting only to be informed there was a two-year waiting list. I thought, 'Two years ago I wasn't even planning a pregnancy!' Securing a nursery spot seemed to be harder than getting tickets to Glastonbury. Luckily, I finally managed to get a place at a nursery where I felt comfortable leaving Georgie.

Leaving your baby with someone else is never going to be a walk in the park, even if it's with family, but especially if it's with strangers. You'll get a gut feeling and I'd strongly recommend visiting a few local places and people before making any decisions or paying any deposits. Most childcare providers recommend an initial 'settling in' period. This is where you accompany your baby to the care provider and support them to familiarise themselves with their new surroundings. This usually takes place over a week or so. Then you'll leave them for an hour and gradually increase.

Feel confident to request what it is you feel your baby needs. If that is more settling in sessions, ask for it. Some babies are happy to go with the flow and settle into new environments smoothly, while others aren't as happy. Remember the evidence about how smell can help (see pages 32–3)? Leaving your baby with something that smells of you may help support them through this transition.

The first time you leave your baby for the day might leave you tearful and worried. Those caring for your baby should have a good understanding of how hard this is for you and respect your need to phone and check or request specific communication arrangements. At Georgie's nursery we have a secure system where her key worker will upload photos and videos of her during the day. Andy and I get updates while she's there, putting both our minds at ease. Find out about the communication tools used by your chosen provider and ensure you are comfortable with them. Your permission should always be sought to take any photos or videos of your child.

Feeling resentful of another caregiver spending precious time with your baby and witnessing things that should be for you to enjoy is a challenge most working mums face. I'm not going to offer a quick fix for these feelings because unfortunately there isn't one. It is hard to accept, but many mums agree it does get easier with time. All changes take time to adapt to – just as it took you time to adapt to becoming a mother, it will take you time to get used to leaving your child with someone else. However, I don't want to mislead you here and brush off a deep gut instinct that serves a purpose. If these feelings do become an issue and things do not gradually get easier, revisit the options above, such as job-sharing, reducing hours, setting up as a freelancer, etc. It's always okay to go back to the drawing board and reconsider if that's what you need to do.

'Naturally, your baby will not want to leave your side when they get home from nursery. That's pretty common, so just set out some time at the end of the day before you start bedtime – even if it's just 15 minutes of sitting and playing or having a cuddle, reading stories together. Just sitting and having that nice time with them to reconnect can be helpful for both of you.'

Laura Smith, specialist community public health nurse (health visitor) Ebonie Chandraraj, specialist community public health nurse (health visitor) @gentlehealthvisitors

RETURNING TO WORK WHILE BREASTFEEDING

Lots of mums ask me about how to return to work and continue feeding. I think it was one of the most common questions popping into my DMs around the time I went back to work.

It's helpful to prepare yourself and your employer for the coming months. If you plan to express at work, you might want to drop your employer an email and explain – among other things or as a separate request. Ask if there is an area that is clean, private and lockable (not a toilet) that can be made available to you, if this is what you want. There is a legal obligation for your employer to provide a place for expressing. How often you will need to express at work will depend on you and your circumstances. The Health and Safety Executive (HSE) provides guidelines and recommendations to protect new mothers at work (see page 243). If you need further help or to encourage your employer to be more flexible, you can consult Maternity Action's website (see page 243) as they provide information and leaflets on maternity and work issues. Hopefully you won't need to refer to any of these, but please feel free to if you're not getting the support you're entitled to.

Lots of mums prefer to start work a little later than they did pre-baby. This is to allow time in the morning to get the both of you ready and fed. Communicating, planning and being as flexible as you can without compromising your needs – yours and your baby's – can help to avoid conflict and stress. The more prepared you are, the less likely you are to feel stressed about returning to work.

Lastly, there's a great template on the Working Families website – the 'Statutory Flexible Working Request Letter' – for you to personalise (see page 244). They've done all the hard work for you, including putting legal requirements in bold. Researching the law and your rights can be time-consuming but copying-and-pasting isn't. Do head there if you'd prefer that option.

Preparing for your return:

- Start to prepare a 'milk bank' of frozen breast milk. A good website containing full details and information on freezing and storing breast milk is La Leche League (see page 242).
- In the weeks before returning to work, have a practice run and organise a routine as if you were already back at work. Make sure your baby's care provider fully understands your plans, safe milk storage/warming, etc. well in advance.
- Try to stick to your usual routine as much as possible, e.g. feeding at 7am – you may need to adapt work hours or your usual morning work routine to fit the feed in.
- If you make sudden or drastic changes, you and your baby will be more aware of these. Small changes, small steps, make things easier in the long run.
- Ensure you make time to pump at work. If you become engorged, you are more at risk of getting blocked ducts or even mastitis (see next page), so ensure you look after yourself. Please never feel guilty for taking the time to pump. It's important for your health!
- Establish a soothing bedtime routine (easier if you don't work nights) and prepare everything for the morning, ensuring your pump and any other necessities are by the door clean and ready so you're not frantically scrabbling about in the morning.

Rest is important and can affect your milk supply – this is the case before and after you return to work. Be prepared to be extra tired in the weeks/months after returning to work, though, as it brings new challenges and considerations. Never, ever feel guilty for resting – this is a unique time in your life and, wherever possible, you need to prioritise your rest.

Try not to worry too much. I know it's easier said than done, but I have been there and worried about things that never happened – we love doing that as mums! Yet babies are resilient and adaptable, and your baby will soon get used to changes, especially if you can remain calm about these changes yourself. Lastly, your baby won't forget how to breastfeed while you're at work; they will reconnect with you and feed as normal when you're reunited. You've got this!

MANAGING MASTITIS

As if the demands of breastfeeding weren't enough, you may also get a blocked milk duct and may then be blessed with the unpleasant infection mastitis, which can present with an array of symptoms: usually feeling fluey, with a visible red patch on your breast, a lump in your breast that you can palpate, pain and raised temperature. I know every trick in the book and I still got it twice. Here are some tips to help manage it:

- Feed through it. So many mums assume it's best to stop, but that worsens it and it's safe to feed through.
- Start feeds with the infected breast.
- Use cooling pads or an ice pack, but remember not to put any ice directly on the skin.
- If your baby is latching well and therefore effectively draining the breast, breastfeeding is usually enough to resolve mastitis. There is no need to pump after a feed in order to empty the breast.
- Avoid wearing a bra if possible – anything digging into your breast will worsen symptoms or perhaps cause another blockage. If you need a bra, opt for non-underwired.
- Drink more than 2 litres of water every day. Flushing out infection works and dehydration can worsen symptoms and the severity of infection.
- Massage your breast to try to gently clear the blockage. Some say to use an electric toothbrush on it if you have one. I don't advise this as it can be too harsh and painful, but it's up to you if you want to give it a go.
- Feed on all fours (this was the bad boy position that cleared mine). It feels odd but lay your baby underneath you and lean over them, dangling your breast in their mouth.

- Speak to your GP if symptoms worsen – you may need a course of antibiotics, but only if you have bacterial mastitis rather than inflammatory. Your GP should be able to differentiate.

If symptoms don't improve within 24 hours, seek medical advice.

STOPPING BREASTFEEDING

When it comes to stopping breastfeeding, as with starting, there are no rules – this is your unique journey. Some babies self-wean or wean off easily, and others are reluctant, protest or even get a bit heavy-handed with you – trying to help themselves. Again, temperament, age, method (baby- or mum-led) or changes in development or at home all impact how they manage their breastfeeding journey coming to a close. By nine months your baby is more able to physically go without milk during the day and to eat food and drink water. But breastmilk is far more than food and is often used by babies and mums as a way of soothing or comforting.

In most cases, weaning is a gradual process unless you need or want to stop abruptly. In this case, you may still need to express to help relieve you and prevent the build-up of milk, which can lead to mastitis (see above).

Here are a few tips to help encourage your baby to wean off the breast:

- Be mindful of associations, such as places you would usually feed – avoid sitting with your baby in a feeding chair.
- Consider your clothing – wearing high-neck tops can help (out of sight/reach encourages out of mind/self-service).
- Shorten feeds gradually.
- Try distractions – maybe a new toy or something at home that's exciting, like a colourful musical instrument. Babies also love stickers – have a sticker party! We had loads!
- Readjust the bedtime routine. It's the bedtime feed that may be the most difficult to drop. Georgie had real trouble dropping that one. It took time. A longer, more drawn-out bedtime routine, patience, and Andy doing bedtime as much as possible got us there in the end – you will get there too.

MANAGING YOUR STRESSOMETER

In general as humans we are resilient. Mothers are another level of strong and we have our grit tested again and again. We will keep getting back up, putting on a brave face and carrying on, pushing ourselves to get through the day, the night and the never-ending to-do list. Our minds and bodies can cope with bursts of stress, but we cannot cope with chronic stress – high levels of stress over a prolonged period of time. We may think we are coping because we are functioning, but it's only a matter of time before we will inevitably become unwell, either physically or mentally. One way to prevent that is regularly checking in with what I like to picture as a stressometer:

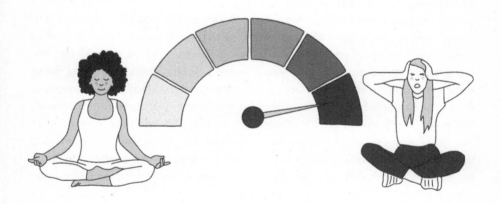

HONESTY BOX

I had to implement this in my life due to my own experience of serious burnout. I went back to work and, although I love the range of work I'm able to do, I didn't carve out *any* time for myself. The requests I received through the Modern Midwife website were flowing quicker than ever. I had some incredible opportunities, such as working with celebrities and big brands; I found myself appearing live on BBC radio channels, being offered keynote speaker slots to large audiences, and I started to get recognised in the street. My career grew significantly more than I could have imagined. But overcommitment and exertion got too much for me. Everything was rushed and I never felt prepared for anything life threw at me. I could not take on what I was used to taking on. The stressometer has worked really well and has given me a little bit of space and time, not much but enough to support my mental health and for me to look after my nervous system a bit better.

At first, check in frequently with the stressometer – as often as every few hours to monitor how you feel. If you're edging towards orange, can you adjust something in that moment or day to help prevent you from reaching red? Each time you creep into the red, no matter what you're doing, STOP. **Avoid remaining in the red at all costs.** Even if it's something for your baby, ensure they're safe but stop what you're doing as soon as you can. As mentioned earlier (see page 145), rushing doesn't usually achieve anything other than the activation of your stress response. So if you too find yourself becoming a frequent rusher, make sure you intervene. Take a deep breath and focus on the out-breath, making it nice and long and deep, ideally three times but if you really don't have the time, just once is better than nothing. That said, there will be times when it's impossible to stop, so when you face those moments make sure you calm your nervous system down after the event and validate your emotions. Have a cuppa, put your hand on you heart and focus on slowing your heart rate, or take some deep, calming breaths before you enter into your next activity or engagement.

Some of the parenting advice I read/watch on Instagram is idealistic and not easy to implement. Setting high expectations can lead to feelings of guilt and self-sabotage if you don't meet them. It's just not always possible and that doesn't mean you're doing anything wrong.

Your best is all you can ever do. Most of us just want to be 'good' parents and do the best for our babies. Simply by having that intention you are on the right path.

I wrote about pacing yourself in labour in my first book and why this is important. Birth can be like a marathon – you don't see marathon runners sprinting at the start for good reason. As a mother myself, I now realise that pacing yourself isn't just for labour, it's for life. Postpartum really is forever. The more you pace yourself and give yourself space the better, keeping in mind the old adage that 'Rome wasn't built in a day' – babies do slow you down and you don't have as much time to do what you did before. That's not because you're failing or inefficient. There's a lot you've got to factor into even the smallest of tasks, like taking a shower. Being a mother to a young baby is a unique time in your life; things gradually get easier as you get used to the calm and knowing the storms do pass.

Happy birthday to you

THERE'S A LOT of pressure around your child's first birthday and you may feel as though you have to throw the biggest party you are able to and get lots of snaps for social media. Give yourself permission to have as big or as small a party as *you* want to. I know we see these extravagant children's birthday parties on Instagram, but what makes a baby happy is not necessarily an aesthetically pleasing birthday. After all, no one actually remembers their first birthday anyway. Take the pressure off yourself and always remember the love you show them on a daily basis is what lasts a lifetime, not the gifts and outward displays.

Someone at work once told me about how they were having a birthday party for themselves as well as their daughter for her first birthday. I did not get it pre-baby, but now I do. You have been through ever so much together in that first year; you've both reached so many milestones and you made it through it all *together*. It is a celebration and one you deserve to enjoy too.

Your life has changed in every way possible and somehow you've coped with the fact that you can't keep everything you had in your life pre-baby. You've made many alterations and amendments and sometimes you've had to drop things, albeit usually temporarily. It's common still to look at other mums with young babies and wonder, 'How do they do it all?' They don't. It may appear that way in the short interaction you have (in the scheme of life), but no one can sustain doing 'it all' – something has to give somewhere once you have a baby. It's okay, it's normal, it happens to us all and you got through it. The things you didn't do or stopped doing aren't holding grudges against you and can be picked up again. I pictured this at the time like physically pressing pause on a remote and looking forward to the day I could press play again. I am pleased to say that, now Georgie is older, I have pressed play on several of those things and you will too. Even if you can't see how right now, it's coming.

Although we didn't throw a separate party, Andy and I did have a celebration afterwards over cocktails and acknowledged what we had been through in that first year as parents. We looked back at photos of us all from her birth and it was a really impactful moment for us as parents. Their first birthday is not just about them – it's about you too and how you got there. After all, your baby has been very dependent on you throughout this year. What an incredible achievement. Happy birthday, mama x

FIRST BIRTHDAY PARTY PLANS

Personally, I think people can go a little over the top these days, but I totally appreciate what a huge milestone you have both reached and why that really deserves a big-time celebration! Again, please don't feel pressure: what you do for your child's birthday is in no way related to how much you care about them.

Here are a few ideas I have seen work well, plus what I did. It doesn't need to be any longer than two hours and make sure you consider the most common nap times. We went for 2–4pm.

Venues
- Local halls: spacious, cheap and supports the local community. (We held Georgie's first birthday at our community hall.)
- Sports centres: these sometimes offer kids' party packages, too.
- Soft play: many offer party packages.
- Your garden, if you have one, or home.

Entertainment ideas
- Kids' entertainer (these can be really reasonably priced).
- Inflatables – or bouncy castle for older kids coming.
- Mini soft play: you can hire these and have them set up anywhere with enough space.
- Food: finger/party food platters you can pick up/order from most supermarkets.
- Music: always a hit with everyone.
- Balloons: again, almost always a hit with kids!

KEY POINTS

- It's likely your baby will be more mobile than ever, either crawling, bum-shuffling or perhaps even walking. Baby-proofing is key to creating a safe environment.
- Behaviours may change that seem to completely throw you. Clinginess can make an appearance again or for the first time – it's part of development at this age.
- Encouraging curiosity and allowing free play to explore helps your baby to problem-solve.
- Career decisions can be tough. It may take you a while to decide or feel comfortable with your decision. Explore all options.
- You may not be able to do the amount or type of things you did before becoming a mum. Let the guilt or judgement fall away. You're doing great.
- Happy birthday to you, mama! The first year is packed with milestones, changes, decisions, difficulties, highs and lows. You got through it all. Go celebrate!

A final note

I HOPE YOU realise just how strong you are and what an incredible job you have done. All mothers really are superwomen. You should be so proud of yourself and the new person you have become. Your resilience, bravery and patience are lifelong skills to carry with you. The pain and hardship you have been through leave a mark on you forever. I really hope my honesty has made you realise you're not alone if you scream into a pillow, feel like you want to run away and hide, or hit rock bottom in your relationship. From the depths of my heart, I send you nothing but love during these times. It's going to be okay.

Remember, your soon-to-be-toddler may challenge you in various other ways as new skill sets emerge over the coming years. Toddlers often want to exercise their right to choose – don't we all? You may find yourself needing to readjust, or even feel a little lost again in the parenting world. It's okay – just like you got this far, you'll get through the next stage. Take each day and each challenge as it comes. Take a breath and give yourself the credit you deserve.

Never worry about how you come across to other people, especially not on social media. You will never be able to please everyone, and the more you try to change yourself to fit the mould of another person's version of 'perfect', the unhappier you will be. By remaining true to your core values and doing your own thing you'll be better able to live authentically. If you're caught in the middle of opinions, you're in limbo – doing what you think other people will think is best rather than following what you really think is best. Following your own instinct as a mother is one of the best things you can do for yourself and your family.

The very last reminder I'd like to leave you with is one of the most important to take with you on your journey. You have the ability to synchronise naturally with your child's brain. This is not something you need actively to try to make happen. It is a natural process that occurs when you're able to just focus on them. A lot of the answers you need, you'll find within yourself, but it can take time to tune in to them. Like looking for a radio station on an old wireless, it's white noise, then, slowly but surely, you hear the clarity of a voice as you fine-tune. Our minds are a little like that – full of thoughts and noise. We need to learn how to quieten the external noise and dial in to ourselves. The answers will almost always come to you if you take a moment to focus with intent.

It's totally okay to make mistakes. Things can be repaired, so forgive yourself, always.

You've got this! x

My top tips

THIS SECTION IS a list of personal reminders that started on my phone, a real-life 'note to self'. This note started to become a bit of a journal in some ways, as I would scramble Georgie back into the car after a play date and quickly type what I had learnt. Or I'd wake up at 5am with her and make a quick note of anything that sprang to mind. Research shows there are wide-ranging benefits of journalling, from reducing anxiety to breaking away from a neurological cycle of obsessive thoughts, improving awareness of things that trigger emotions, gaining a better perception of events to help with regulating emotions, and boosting physical health – even the immune system.

After overcoming a tough time, I always found I learnt something and wanted to keep a log to help remind myself of these for the next tough phase, or when guilt would show up. These notes have helped me self-soothe and put things into perspective. To make them more relevant to you, I have slightly changed the wording (and removed a few swear words – feel free to mentally insert where you feel applicable!). I hope you too find these useful, and I'd really encourage you to start a little note on your phone as an outlet and way of reminding yourself of your unique journey through motherhood. You really are superwoman.

Below is a QR code for you to scan that takes you to a digital copy of the notes listed here, which will be updated regularly. Like me, you may find it useful to have these to hand when you're out and about, or getting through a 3am feed.

- **Parent yourself before any of your children.** We may see advice from just about every parenting expert that focuses on how best to care for our kids, but our parenting ability (or limits) often start with self-care (or lack of it). In order to be the best version of yourself, the mother you want to be, you need to speak to yourself with love, care, self-compassion and understanding. Parenting will challenge you and your limits in every way possible. You're going to be okay and work through this huge learning curve and transition.

- **Motherhood is like being in a time machine** – never before has time gone so fast yet so slowly. The days are long, but the years are short. Things you remember as though they were yesterday end up being many months back. Take as many videos and photos as you can, and ask other people to do this for you so you can really be present in the moment and physically in the photos.

- **Nurture *their* nature.** Every child is different, just like every adult. If you have more than one child, you'll very quickly realise you need to adapt your parenting to their needs rather than the other way around. They are who *they* are. That is why it's important to get to know *your* baby. Although expert advice may be helpful, nothing will ever trump how well you know your baby. Try to look inwards before seeking external advice and following any advice that doesn't feel right for you. Feel free to brush it off, keep your chin up, and have confidence.

- **Try not to take crying personally.** It's a lot easier said than done. Georgie just turned two years old and I have to remind myself of this regularly. Crying or even screaming is a baby's only form of communication for a long time. Babies under six months usually need something fixing/feeding/changing, etc. Older babies will also 'cry for need', but sometimes they just 'need to cry'. There will be a day (or several) when you go through everything you can to fix it for them, or offer solutions, and still they cry. Know that it's not because you're a bad mum. Sometimes they need to cry and release emotion. Especially as they get older. I first see if I can fix why she's crying and, if not, I allow her emotion to come to the surface, offer her a cuddle or security, and let her work through it.

- **Everything is worse at night.** Everything! Your tolerance and their discomfort. From a bit of nappy rash to a tooth erupting. There are no distractions after dark and you're exhausted – willing to do almost anything to get some sleep. Your patience may wear thinner than ever overnight. The sun will rise and you will get through those dark nights and moments. Make sure you ask for help the following day, and go *very* easy on yourself. It's okay (in fact preferable) to cancel a class or lunch date if you need to and nap with your baby, or sit in your PJs and recover from the stress.

HONESTY BOX

I clearly remember one night with Georgie, after five months of sleep deprivation, this one night was the worst night of our lives so far. She cried on and off all night until 5am. By then I felt like my world was ending. I wasn't even a person let alone a mother. I went into the garden (mid-Jan) in a T-shirt and my massive Bridget Jones knickers to do some deep breathing when I heard her start crying again. I didn't have it in me to go back inside straight away. I finished my deep breathing and let her cry for a minute. I was at the end of my tether and had lost all ability to function. That day we had plans, but instead I didn't shower or get changed. I sat with the TV on, ate chocolate cake and allowed myself to rest as much as possible and recuperate. It's okay to put yourself first – especially if that preserves your mental health.

- **You may not be an expert in child development, but you are an expert in your baby.** Always remember that and if your intuition tells you something, follow it. Mother's intuition is a really powerful one and the bond you two have is greater than any amount of expertise. You know your child, so have confidence in that knowledge.
- **Just when you think you've nailed it, it all changes.** Try not to focus on the disruption of the change and instead focus on what you can do to go with it or how you can adapt. Always far easier said than done and I still very much have to remind myself of this. It's easy to get caught up in the emotions associated with change and the confusion, but the best use of your limited energy is to accept and move with the change. Unless it's a change you're not willing to accept, of course. Usually phases pass, but you may want to approach these situations differently and implement boundaries.
- **What may seem like the biggest issue you're facing right now will soon be a memory** or sometimes even un-rememberable. They're soon on to the next phase and it all happens so fast: 'This too shall pass.'
- **Babies are not born with the capacity to understand movement and predict its consequences.** They have to learn this, which is why

they often love dropping items on the floor or observing movement. Encourage or allow this where possible because it's a part of their development – hugely annoying though it can be to be forever picking up the toy they love dropping.

- **Our brains exist to drive behaviour and to take in information from the world and act accordingly.** One of the most important things for us to teach our babies is how to belong in the context of the world in which they live. Considering what is important where they are growing up, how can you improve their understanding of this time and day and age? Applying your history or how you were parented may not be applicable or at all relevant to them. Have the confidence to recognise that and parent in a way you feel is effective for raising your child in the context of their time.

- **You won't always get it right and that's okay.** Instead, you'll learn, grow and change. Forgive yourself for the times you get it wrong and move on quickly. If possible, recognise and own your mistakes – we are human and we all make them. You can only ever do your best given your circumstances. Redemption is powerful.

- **The more honest you are with other mums, the stronger you'll feel.** Keeping things – feelings, struggles and frustrations – to yourself can lead to feelings of loneliness. I am sure that anything you have struggled with I likely have too, and if not me, then another mum certainly will have. Anyone who judges you for being honest is not your friend. Harsh but true. The very last thing you need is judgement. You'll likely do enough of that to yourself. You need to be able to open up and bond over the shared hardships. I have a very good friend, Michelle, and although we experience different things, she has not once judged me. She listens, validates and offers potential solutions. Sometimes she just listens and comforts me without trying to fix things. Find your Michelle; she'll change your mum life.

HONESTY BOX

I was a massive people pleaser. I would put myself out for other people, drag myself to events/parties I really didn't want to go to, and rarely ever said what I really thought – for fear of upsetting those around me. I have come to realise that some of those traits, although coming from a good place, are damaging. I would let my friends buy me things I hated because I didn't tell them right away. I'd end up in situations I didn't want to be in, wishing I had said no to begin with. People would occasionally mistake my kindness for weakness and take advantage of me. I would finally notice this and then erupt. I'd suppressed my own needs and feelings superficially but they were there, deep in my core. And my goodness did they show up eventually. Erupting is not cool or pleasant, and achieves a whole lot of nothing. It's often the result of people-pleasing, though. The more you try to please everyone, the more unhappy you become because you're not able to live authentically. This is a generalisation, but people are easily offended these days, making the people pleasers feel even more on edge. If people don't like you for being yourself, maybe it's time to question if they really are 'your people'. Motherhood can be a great time to implement less people-pleasing and more authentic living. For you and your whole family. You've got this.

'If you find yourself in a friendship group that makes you feel worse, it's probably time to find a new village, or not necessarily fall out with those people but find the ones to spend time with who make you feel good. Also, sometimes you are parenting differently to how your parents or grandparents did, and you can feel undermined, or they can make you feel bad or that you're doing something wrong. Find other mums whose values are a bit more aligned with yours. It's not about falling out with other people but just finding those who are going to support you in that period of your life.'

Laura Smith, specialist community public health nurse (health visitor) Ebonie Chandraraj, specialist community public health nurse (health visitor) @gentlehealthvisitors

- **New mothers need to be mothered.** I love the saying 'The nurturer needs to be nurtured' because it's so very true. Although the self-care bandwagon has been drummed up for a long time, or maybe misrepresented, it's always worth promoting in motherhood. As I've mentioned, self-care looks very different for different people, and caring for you, as early into motherhood as possible and as often as possible, is a crucial part of promoting good mental health and self-compassion.

- **Guilt will show up in your life.** Likely more than ever before. Allow the emotion, sit with it, find out what it's teaching you and try to let it go. Every mum feels guilty about something. We can't avoid it, but what we can do is be compassionate towards ourselves when it does show up and remind ourselves that no human walking the earth is perfect. They never have been and never will be. You're doing amazing.

- **Becoming a mother yourself may lead to feelings of need to be with or near your own mum.** Conversely, it can also bring up feelings of resentment towards your own mother – depending on your upbringing and any differences over your parenting styles. Either one is a natural response to this shift in your life as you walk into the world of motherhood yourself. Yet again, notice how you feel, try to address it and, if you're able to, speak to someone you trust about your feelings.

- **An identity crisis can be tough.** Who are you? Are your dreams, goals and any aspirations you have falling by the wayside? Is the person you were pre-baby still there? These questions and more are hard to answer, but they do not need intervention. Sometimes life unfolds and we take a different path; we pause on our path and later continue, or we stop altogether. All of these are okay. There's no rush to 'get back' and you can't force time to pass. It's best to accept where you are in your life at this time.

Helpful resources

For evidence-based posts and a big dose of reality, you can head to my website or Instagram:

https://www.themodernmidwife.com

@the_modern_midwife

For anything you're really concerned about you can always go to A&E. Call your midwife or GP or 111 for anything less urgent or concerning.

Babywearing

For more on how to safely carry your baby and research on the benefits, see the following resources:

Carrying Matters

https://www.carryingmatters.co.uk/sling-pages

ROSPA

https://www.rospa.com/home-safety/advice/product/baby-slings

UK Sling Consortium

http://babyslingsafety.co.uk

Birthing experiences

Support for any of your concerns around birth.

Birthing Awareness

https://birthingawarenesstraining.com

Birth Trauma Association

Support for women who have had a traumatic birth experience; offers emotional and practical support to those suffering post-traumatic stress disorder, and their families. It has a Facebook support group.

https://birthtraumaassociation.org.uk

Make Birth Better

https://www.makebirthbetter.org

Breast- and bottle-feeding

If you need help with breast- or bottle-feeding, talk to your midwife or health visitor or call the helplines below:

La Leche League

Offers breastfeeding support and information.

See https://www.laleche.org.uk/get-support for your local helpline or call the national line on 0345 120 2918

National Childbirth Trust (NCT)

The NCT gives practical and emotional support with bottle-feeding or breast-feeding your baby, and can help with any concerns or questions.

Call 0300 330 0700, daily, 8am–midnight, or go to https://www.nct.org.uk

UK National Breastfeeding Helpline

Run by the Breastfeeding Network and the Association of Breastfeeding Mothers, volunteers on the end of the line are mums who have breastfed and have been trained in giving breastfeeding support.

Call 0300 100 0212, 9.30am–9.30pm daily

Live online service is also available at www.nationalbreastfeedinghelpline.org.uk

Crying

CRY-SIS

Helpline for advice: 0800 448 0737 (9am–10pm, seven days a week)

https://www.cry-sis.org.uk

Domestic abuse

National Domestic Abuse Helpline

0808 2000 247

https://www.nationaldahelpline.org.uk

Refuge

https://refuge.org.uk

Women's Aid

https://www.womensaid.org.uk

Eating disorders
Beat

Supporting people who have battled eating disorders in the past or are in need of a diagnosis.

https://www.beateatingdisorders.org.uk

Family planning
Fertility UK

https://www.fertilityuk.org

First aid
Resuscitation Council

https://www.resus.org.uk

Health
Healthier Together

https://www.what0-18.nhs.uk

NHS

https://www.nhs.uk/conditions

https://www.nhs.uk/conditions/vaccinations/nhs-vaccinations-and-when-to-have-them

Maternity and workplace guidelines
HSE (Health and Safety Executive)

https://www.hse.gov.uk/mothers

Maternity Action

Provides information and leaflets on maternity and work issues.

https://maternityaction.org.uk/know-your-rights

Working Families

You can get free legal advice by calling the Working Families hotline on 0300 012 0312

There's also a 'Statutory Flexible Working Request' letter template for you to personalise on their website:

https://workingfamilies.org.uk/articles/sample-letter-to-request-flexible-working

Mental health
Your GP and health visitor can help, as well as the charities below.

Action on Postpartum Psychosis (APP)

Offers a peer support network online, including one-to-one support.

https://www.app-network.org

Anna Mathur

Psychotherapist and author Anna Mathur shares a lot of free advice online.

https://www.annamathur.com

The Association for Post Natal Illness

Provides support for mums suffering from postnatal illness. Volunteers have experienced and recovered from postnatal illness.

Call 0207 386 0868, 10am–2pm Monday to Friday, or use the online chat box at: https://apni.org

Maternal OCD

A charity that provides information and support to mums experiencing peri-natal obsessive-compulsive disorder (OCD).

For peer support email info@maternalocd.org or see https://maternalocd.org for a list of further resources.

PANDAS Foundation

Provides support and advice for any parent experiencing perinatal mental illness.

Call 0808 1961 776, 11am–10pm daily, or see https://pandasfoundation.org.uk

Multiple births
Twins Trust

https://twinstrust.org

Single parenting
Gingerbread

Call 0808 802 0925 (check website for hours)

https://www.gingerbread.org.uk

Sleep
Basis

Baby sleep information.

https://www.basisonline.org.uk

The Lullaby Trust

https://www.lullabytrust.org.uk

See also The Lullaby Trust Baby Check app, which can help parents or carers determine how ill their baby is. Available free from Google Play or the App Store: https://www.lullabytrust.org.uk/safer-sleep-advice/baby-check-app

Please use these links for further information on the following:

- When babies start to roll: https://www.lullabytrust.org.uk/safer-sleep-advice/sleeping-position
- Premature babies: https://www.lullabytrust.org.uk/safer-sleep-advice/premature-babies
- Baby boxes: https://www.lullabytrust.org.uk/wp-content/uploads/baby-box-info-leaflet.pdf

Support for women
Mums Anywhere

https://mumsanywhere.com

Mush

@mushmums on Instagram

Peanut

https://www.peanut-app.io

Weaning

Charlotte Stirling-Reed

Charlotte is an award-winning baby and child nutritionist, and has some brilliant free advice and resources on weaning on her website, as well as books, workshops and online courses.

https://www.srnutrition.co.uk

Recommended TED Talk

Vilayanur Ramachandran, 'The neurons that shaped civilization'

References

PART 1: THE FIRST 48 HOURS AFTER BIRTH

Wounds and bleeding

Assessment and repair of any wounds: 'There are very small and simple things that you can do to prevent perineal trauma, such as the choice of your place of birth (research shows that mums who give birth in a midwifery-led unit or at home have significantly reduced chances of perineal trauma).'

Kurinczuk, J.J., Knight, M., Rowe, R. and Hollowell, J., *Evidence Review to Support the National Maternity Review 2015; Report 1: Summary of the evidence on safety of place of birth; and implications for policy and practice from the overall evidence review* (National Perinatal Epidemiology Unit, University of Oxford, 2015)

Birth experiences

A long labour: 'According to researchers, a person who feels that their emotions are not wrong or inappropriate is more likely to have a solid sense of identity and worth and can manage emotions more effectively.'

Westphal, M., Leahy, R.L., Pala, A.N. and Wupperman, P., 'Self-compassion and emotional invalidation mediate the effects of parental indifference on psychopathology', *Psychiatry Research* 242 (2016): https://doi.org/10.1016/j.psychres.2016.05.040

'The charity Birth Trauma Association estimates that 30,000 women suffer with birth trauma in the UK alone, every year.'

Heyne, C.S. et al., 'Prevalence and risk factors of birth-related posttraumatic stress among parents: a comparative systematic review and meta-analysis', *Clinical Psychology Review* 94 (2022): https://doi.org/10.1016/j.cpr.2022.102157

Caring for your mental health after birth: 'In the UK, up to 20 per cent of mums are diagnosed with postnatal depression (PND), and suicide remains the leading cause of death for mums in the perinatal period (during pregnancy and the year following birth).'

https://maternalmentalhealthalliance.org/news/mbrrace-suicide-leading-cause-maternal-death

Meeting your newborn

The importance of smell: 'Ruth Feldman, Simms-Mann Professor of Developmental Social Neuroscience at the Interdisciplinary Center (IDC) Herzliya, Israel, wanted to find out more.'

Feldman, R. et al., 'Maternal chemosignals enhance infant-adult brain-to-brain synchrony', *Science Advances* 7(50) (2023): https://www.science.org/doi/10.1126/sciadv.abg6867

Admission to Neonatal Intensive Care Unit (NICU): 'According to the World Health Organization (WHO), globally 15 million babies are born prematurely every year; 60 per cent of these births take place in Africa and South Asia. Around 1 in 13 babies are born prematurely in the UK.'

https://www.who.int/news-room/fact-sheets/detail/preterm-birth

Feeding your baby

Breastfeeding and realistic expectations: 'After all, NHS Digital reports that around 74 per cent of mums initiate breastfeeding.'

https://digital.nhs.uk/data-and-information/publications/statistical/maternity-services-monthly-statistics

Setting yourself up: 'Women are not to be blamed or shamed for this; instead, we need to look at what we are doing differently to countries like Croatia, where there's a staggering 82.7 per cent breastfeeding rate.'

https://www.unicef.org/croatia/en/baby-friendly-maternity-wards

Responsive breastfeeding: '"Responsive breastfeeding involves a mother responding to her baby's cues, as well as her own desire to feed her baby. Crucially, feeding responsively recognises that feeds are not just for nutrition, but also for love, comfort and reassurance between baby and mother."'

https://www.unicef.org.uk/babyfriendly/wp-content/uploads/sites/2/2017/12/Responsive-Feeding-Infosheet-Unicef-UK-Baby-Friendly-Initiative.pdf

'I don't have enough milk': 'Perceived insufficient milk supply is the major reason mums stop breastfeeding.'

Huang, Y. et al., 'The rates and factors of perceived insufficient milk supply: a systematic review', *Maternal and Child Nutrition* 18(1) (2021): https://onlinelibrary.wiley.com/doi/full/10.1111/mcn.13255

Formula-feeding: 'As we know, in the UK 99 per cent of babies will receive some formula milk by six months, whether that's in combination with breast milk or on its own.'

https://www.bpas.org/get-involved/campaigns/briefings/breastfeeding-and-formula-feeding

PART 2: NEWBORN TO THREE MONTHS

The first 42 days

'Roughly 38 per cent of women diagnosed with PND found it becomes a lifelong condition, according to a report published in the *Harvard Review of Psychiatry* in 2014.'

Vliegen, N., Casalin, S. and Lutyen, P., 'The course of postpartum depression: a review of longitudinal studies', *Harvard Review of Psychiatry* 22(1) (2014): https://doi.org/10.1097/HRP.0000000000000013

'Another Australian study showed that the peak incidence of depression postnatally was shockingly around four to five years after the birth of a baby. This is possibly due to changing support as babies become children, as well as recurring mental health symptoms that become progressively worse over time.'

Bryson, H. et. al., 'Patterns of maternal depression, anxiety, and stress symptoms from pregnancy to 5 years postpartum in an Australian cohort experiencing adversity', *Archives of Women's Mental Health* 24(6) (2021): https://www.ncbi.nlm.nih.gov/pmc/articles/PMC8148407/

Common symptoms

Can pregnancy help us understand long-term health?: 'The physiological changes and symptoms you experience could therefore be early indicators of potential predispositions to certain health conditions.'

Duley, L. 'The global impact of pre-eclampsia and eclampsia'. *Semin. Perinatol.* 33, 130–137 (2009)

Haemorrhoids (piles): 'Please try not to feel embarrassed or worried about them – they're common and it's estimated that around 40 per cent of women experience them.'

Bužinskienė, D. et. al., 'Perianal diseases in pregnancy and after childbirth: frequency, risk factors, impact on women's quality of life and treatment methods', *Frontiers in Surgery* 9 (2022): https://doi.org/10.3389/fsurg.2022.788823

The six-week postnatal check: 'NHS Blood and Transplant report up to 41 per cent of postnatal mothers become anaemic.'

https://www.rcpath.org/profession/publications/college-bulletin/july-2021/anaemia-in-pregnancy-and-the-postpartum-period.html

Hair loss: 'We can't be certain this is related to humans, but high cortisol levels in sheep are associated with increased postpartum hair loss.'

Taha, R., 'Hematological, biochemical and hormonal studies on postpartum alopecia in ewes', *Journal of American Science* 8(9) (2012):https://doi.org/10.7537/marsjas080912.133

Increased noise sensitivity: 'One study found that, after birth, tissue increases within auditory areas.'

Luders, E. et al., 'Postpartum gray matter changes in the auditory cortex', *Journal of Clinical Medicine* 10(23) (2021): https://doi.org/10.3390/jcm10235616

'Another study found that high levels of emotional exhaustion increase sound sensitivity.'

Hasson, D. et al., 'Acute stress induces hyperacusis in women with high levels of emotional exhaustion', *PLOS One* 8(1) (2013): https://www.ncbi.nlm.nih.gov/pmc/articles/PMC3534646/

Mental health in the fourth trimester

Gossips: 'Mothers had a group of women around them, consisting of the midwife and the "gossips".'

Briffett, E. 'Where does the word 'gossip' come from – and what has it got to do with childbirth?' *History Extra*, 14 March 2022: https://www.historyextra.com/period/general-history/gossip-why-do-we-say-childbirth-meaning/

Safer sleep for babies

Making the decision to co-sleep: 'One study published by the American Academy of Sleep Medicine concluded [. . .]'

Fuentes, B., 'Bed sharing versus sleeping alone associated with sleep health and mental health', *Sleep* 45(1) (2022): https://doi.org/10.1093/sleep/zsac079.009

'Henning Johannes Drews, a researcher at the Center for Integrative Psychiatry and a professor at the Department of Psychiatry and Psychotherapy at Christian-Albrechts University, Kiel, Germany, studied 12 heterosexual couples who spent four nights in a sleep lab – not a large sample size, but still really interesting to study.'

Drews, H.J. et al., '"Are we in sync with each other?" Exploring the effects of cosleeping on heterosexual couples' sleep using simultaneous polysomnography: a pilot study', *Sleep Disorders* (2017): https://pubmed.ncbi.nlm.nih.gov/28465841/

Supporting your baby's development

The impact of separation: 'Research by the World Health Organization shows that COVID-19 severely affected the care given to small and sick newborns, resulting in unnecessary suffering and loss.'

https://www.who.int/news/item/16-03-2021-new-research-highlights-risks-of-separating-newborns-from-mothers-during-covid-19-pandemic

'A study published in the *Lancet*'s *eClinicalMedicine* highlights the critical importance of ensuring newborn babies have very close contact with parents after birth, especially for those born small (at low birth weight) or prematurely.'

Minckas, N. et al., 'Preterm care during the COVID-19 pandemic: a comparative risk analysis of neonatal deaths averted by kangaroo mother care versus mortality due to SARS-CoV-2 infection', *eClinicalMedicine* 33(100733) (2021): https://doi.org/10.1016/j.eclinm.2021.100733

Eye contact, talking and singing: 'Anthropologists too have written about the anxiety-reducing effects of singing, praying or crying together.'

Gračanin, A., Bylsma, L.M. and Vingerhoets, A.J.J.M., 'Is crying a self-soothing behavior?', *Frontiers in Psychology* 5 (2014): https://www.ncbi.nlm.nih.gov/pmc/articles/PMC4035568/

'Two Harvard Medical School researchers found that singing lullabies to infants helped to soothe and calm them when crying or distressed.'

https://medicalxpress.com/news/2018-03-lullabies-concerts-music-rhythm-social.html

https://news.harvard.edu/gazette/story/2017/03/why-sing-to-baby-because-if-you-dont-youll-starve/

Baby signing: 'Although initially babies who learn to sign may be better communicators, researchers found that when babies were 30 months and 36 months old there was no statistically significant difference between groups.'

Goodyear, S.W., Acredolo, L.P. and Brown, C.A., 'Impact of symbolic gesturing on early language', *Journal of Nonverbal Behavior* 24(2) (2000): https://doi.org/10.1023/A:1006653828895

Play and movement: 'Newborn babies are capable of making conscious movement and this has been proven when studied.'

van der Meer, A.L.H. and van der Weel, F.R.R., 'The optical information for self-perception in development'. In Wagman, J.B. and Blau, J.C. Blau (Eds.), *Perception as Information Detection: Reflections on Gibson's Ecological Approach to Visual Perception* (pp. 110-129). Routledge/Taylor and Francis (2020).

Crying

Crying and human rituals: 'There is a fascinating piece of research into adult rituals, comforting behaviours and infant crying that I recently read up on.'

Gračanin, A., Bylsma, L.M., Vingerhoets, A.J., 'Is crying a self-soothing behavior?', *Frontiers in Psychology* 5 (2014): https://doi.org/10.3389/fpsyg.2014.00502

Top tips for dummy usage: 'Some research suggests they may reduce the risk of SIDS.'

https://www.nhs.uk/conditions/baby/caring-for-a-newborn/reduce-the-risk-of-sudden-infant-death-syndrome/#:~:text=It%27s%20possible%20using%20a%20dummy,is%20around%201%20month%20old

Colic: 'Studies have shown that 20 per cent of infants cry for long periods without any apparent reason during the first four months.'

St James-Roberts, I., Alvarez, M. and Hovish, K., 'Emergence of a developmental explanation for prolonged crying in 1- to 4-month-old infants: review of the evidence', *Journal of Pediatric Gastroenterology and Nutrition* 57(1):S30–S36 (2013) http://doi.org/10.1097/01.mpg.0000441932.07469.1b

'Causes of colic are often unknown; however, guidelines from the National Institute for Health and Care Excellence (NICE) and the NHS Choices website both suggest that some babies may have short-term problems with digesting lactose (a natural milk sugar found in breast and formula milk).'

https://www.nhs.uk/common-health-questions/childrens-health/what-should-i-do-if-i-think-my-baby-is-allergic-or-intolerant-to-cows-milk/

https://cks.nice.org.uk/topics/cows-milk-allergy-in-children/

Jaundice: 'Around 60 per cent of babies become jaundiced within the first week of life; it rarely starts before 24 hours and usually self-resolves in ten days.'

https://www.england.nhs.uk/wp-content/uploads/2015/07/jaundice-in-the-newborn.pdf

PART 3: THREE TO SIX MONTHS

What to expect

Trying to communicate with you: 'Research shows that mirroring supports bonding and attachment, but also aids development.'

Rayson, H. et al., 'Early maternal mirroring predicts infant motor system activation during facial expression observation', *Scientific Reports* 7(1), (2017): https://www.nature.com/articles/s41598-017-12097-w

Improved motor skills: 'According to Dr Kang Lee at the Dr. Erick Jackman Institute of Child Study, University of Toronto [. . .]'

Lee, K. et al., 'Older but not younger infants associate own-race faces with happy music and other-race faces with sad music', *Developmental Science* 21(2) (2018): https://onlinelibrary.wiley.com/doi/full/10.1111/desc.12537

What's happening with your baby

Brain-to-brain synchrony: 'Professor Rebecca Saxe, a cognitive neuroscientist from the United States, was one of the first scientists in human history to undertake an MRI scan on a nine-week-old baby – her son Arthur – and then again on her second baby, Percy, aged three months at the time.'

https://neurosciencenews.com/neuroimaging-baby-neurodevelopment-5914/

'Research has also proved something most of us may have guessed: that multi-sensory stimulation supports healthy brain development in babies.'

https://www.ncbi.nlm.nih.gov/pmc/articles/PMC3722610/

Teething: 'Here's a rough guide from the NHS to how babies' teeth usually emerge [. . .]'

https://www.nhs.uk/conditions/baby/babys-development/teething/baby-teething-symptoms/

Relationship difficulties

'One study included 218 couples spanning the first eight years of marriage and concluded that parenthood significantly impacts marital function.'

Doss, B. D. et al., 'The effect of the transition to parenthood on relationship quality: an eight-year prospective study', *Journal of Personality and Social Psychology* 96(3): https://www.ncbi.nlm.nih.gov/pmc/articles/PMC2702669/

The overload for modern mums: 'Not only do I hear this anecdotally on a regular basis, but it's reflected in statistics from the Office for National Statistics [. . .]'

https://www.ons.gov.uk/employmentandlabourmarket/peopleinwork/employmentandemployeetypes/articles/familiesandthelabourmarketengland/2021#:~:text=1.-,Main%20points,(66.5%25%20in%202002)

Taking ownership: 'Research shows that the majority of parents argue more during the first year than at any other time, so we weren't unusual.'

https://www.apa.org/monitor/2011/10/babies

PART 4: SIX TO NINE MONTHS

What to expect

The need to nap: 'One study found that having an extended nap of 30 minutes or more within four hours of learning a set of object–action pairings from a puppet toy enabled six- and 12-month-old infants to retain their memories of new behaviour.'

Tham, E.K., Schneider, N. and Broekman, B.F., 'Infant sleep and its relation with cognition and growth: a narrative review', *Nature and Science of Sleep* 9 (2017): https://doi.org/10.2147/NSS.S125992

Weaning

'The UK charity Beat (formerly Eating Disorders Association) estimates that around 1.25 million people in the UK have an eating disorder – with 75 per cent of those affected being female.'

https://www.beateatingdisorders.org.uk/media-centre/eating-disorder-statistics/

When is the best time to start weaning?: 'The NHS, the Department of Health and the WHO recommend weaning a baby at around six months.Yet research by the Office for Health Improvement and Disparities (OHID) found that 40 per cent of first-time mums introduce solid food by the time their baby is five months old and almost two-thirds (64 per cent) say they have received conflicting advice on the best age to start weaning.'

https://www.gov.uk/government/news/new-campaign-promotes-advice-to-introduce-babies-to-solid-food

'The OHID states: "The introduction of solid foods may reduce the amount of breast milk consumed and is associated with greater risks of infectious illness in infants. Giving solid foods to breastfed infants before six months may also reduce breast milk intake without increasing total energy intake or increasing weight gain."'

https://www.gov.uk/government/news/new-campaign-promotes-advice-to-introduce-babies-to-solid-food

How do babies taste food before they're born?: 'The "carrot juice experiment" involved mums who drank carrot juice in pregnancy and mums who drank carrot juice in the first two months of breastfeeding.'

Menella, J.A., Jagnow, C.P. and Beauchamp, G.K., 'Prenatal and postnatal flavor learning by human infants', *Pediatrics* 107(6) (2001): https://www.ncbi.nlm.nih.gov/pmc/articles/PMC1351272/

How to wean: 'Research suggests that the period of six to nine months is when babies are most accepting of new foods (referred to as the "window of opportunity").'

Borowitz, S.M., 'First Bites – Why, when, and what solid foods to feed infants', *Frontiers in Pediatrics* 9 (2021): https://www.ncbi.nlm.nih.gov/pmc/articles/PMC8032951/

'The research demonstrates that this approach can have a positive impact on vegetable intake.'

Johnson, S.L., 'Developmental and environmental influences on young children's vegetable preferences and consumption', *Advances in Nutrition* 7(1) (2016): https://www.ncbi.nlm.nih.gov/pmc/articles/PMC4717879/

'The NHS also states that it's important not to offer babies and young children salt or salty foods (which includes bacon and sausages); sugar or sugary snacks; foods high in saturated fats; mould-ripened or blue-veined soft cheeses, ripened goat's milk cheese or cheeses made from unpasteurised milk; raw and lightly cooked eggs; rice drinks; raw jelly cubes; raw shellfish; or fish high in mercury, such as shark, marlin or swordfish.'

https://www.nhs.uk/conditions/baby/weaning-and-feeding/foods-to-avoid-giving-babies-and-young-children/

Gut health for babies: 'An interesting study found there is a difference in the composition of bacteria for babies born via C-section compared to vaginal birth.'

Coelho, G.D.P. et al., 'Acquisition of microbiota according to the type of birth: an integrative review', *Revista Latino-Americana de Enfermagem* 29 (2021): https://www.ncbi.nlm.nih.gov/pmc/articles/PMC8294792/

'So much so that research has revealed there is very little difference in gut health in babies born via C-section if breastfed for six months after birth.'

https://www.newscientist.com/article/2363496-breastfed-c-section-babies-get-more-of-their-microbiomes-from-milk/

There is also some research into how pets (impartially, dogs) support gut health by leading to a more diverse microbiome.'

Panzer, A.R. et al., 'The impact of prenatal dog keeping on infant gut microbiata development', *Clinical & Experimental Allergy* (2023): https://doi.org/10.1111/cea.14303

'Research has shown that probiotic supplements may lessen the impact of antibiotics on a baby's gut microbiome, so this is worth discussing with your GP.'

Johnston, B.C. et al., 'Probiotics for the prevention of pediatric antibiotic-associated diarrhea', *Cochrane Database of Systematic Reviews* (2019): https://pubmed.ncbi.nlm.nih.gov/22071814/

PART 5: NINE TO TWELVE MONTHS

~~~~~

What to expect

Curiosity drives learning: 'He decided to run a very interesting experiment which highlighted the importance of curiosity to the learning process.'

Oudeyer, P.-Y. and Smith, L.B., 'How evolution may work through curiosity-driven developmental process', *Topics in Cognitive Science* 8(2) (2016): https://pubmed.ncbi.nlm.nih.gov/26969919/

Putting your needs first

'The largest population-based study to date found that 17.22 per cent of mothers globally suffered with PND, equating to millions of mothers every single year.'

Wang, Z. et al., 'Mapping global prevalence of depression among postpartum women', *Translational Psychiatry* 11 (2021): https://www.ncbi.nlm.nih.gov/pmc/articles/PMC8528847/

Going back to work (or not)

Wanting to return to work: 'A 2018 study published by the Business Performance Innovation Network found that 63 per cent of parents who work outside the home have experienced some form of parental burnout.'

https://www.bpinetwork.org/thought-leadership/studies/67

My Top Tips

'Research shows there are wide-ranging benefits of journalling, from reducing anxiety to breaking away from a neurological cycle of obsessive thoughts, improving awareness of things that trigger emotions, gaining a better perception of events to help with regulating emotions, and boosting physical health – even the immune system.'

Smyth, J.M et al., 'Online positive affect journaling in the improvement of mental distress and well-being in general medical patients with elevated anxiety symptoms: a preliminary randomized controlled trial', *JMIR Mental Health* 5(4) (2018): https://www.ncbi.nlm.nih.gov/pmc/articles/PMC6305886/

https://positivepsychology.com/benefits-of-journaling/

About the author

Marie Louise is a midwife, adult educator, hypnobirthing teacher and author of the bestselling *The Modern Midwife's Guide to Pregnancy, Birth and Beyond*. You can find her on Instagram @the_modern_midwife or at themodernmidwife.com for informative and evidence-based guidance.

Acknowledgements

Never in my wildest dreams did I think I was capable of writing not one but two books. You would not be reading this if it wasn't for the incredible people I am so fortunate to have in my life. There's no way this book would have been possible without them.

There are so many people who have supported me on this journey and I'd really like to take a moment to thank them.

Firstly, my darling Georgie, you are the light and love of my life. As you know, you've taught me so much about myself, the world and what true love really is. I do not know who I would be without you. You're the reason I decided to write this book. I will always be with you.

Andy, my partner in life. Thank you for supporting me to be the woman I am. For hearing me out when I needed to vent and for sticking by me in our toughest times. No matter what, we will always be a team. Thank you for letting me share so much of us in this book.

My family, my mum, dad, brother and sister. I miss you every day now we live so far apart but your cheering on and constant reassurance always drive me forward and keep me on track. Both personally and professionally. I love you all so much and you made me the mother and author I can now call myself.

Natalie Collins, my amazing assistant. Thank you for always having my back, reading the first draft of the first chapter and always being so open and honest with me. Thank you for taking some of the pressure off me and giving me the space I needed to write.

Jason Foo and your introduction to the amazing Helen Tupper. Your consistent guidance and support made this book (and many of my career successes) happen. I will never know how to thank you. Eternally grateful.

Every contributor in the book. Your expertise and guidance have been such a great comfort and I have learnt a lot from you all during the course of writing this book. Thank you for giving up your time to support parents and for being so dedicated to your field of work. You're making such an impact.

Sam Jackson, for once again believing in me more than I believed in myself and making this book happen. And Julia Kellaway, my 'wizard' editor. Thank you for shaping and making this book what it is. The book needed you so much. I hope there's a third and we work together again!

Lastly to you, the reader, also known as 'mama'. Thank you for taking the time to buy this book, read it and spend time with me. Your time is precious but I really hope you feel supported and that this book normalises your struggles and juggles.

Index

Note: page numbers in **bold** refer to illustrations.